Sai Ashtang Yoga

Pathway to Self Realisation

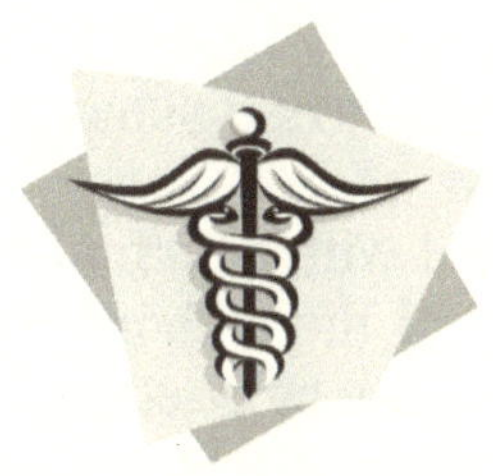

Dr. Kavita S. Bhatt

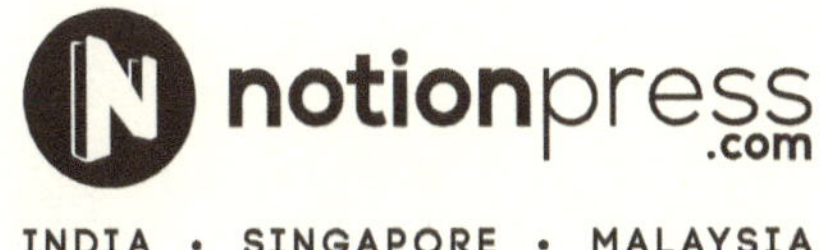

notionpress
.com

INDIA • SINGAPORE • MALAYSIA

ISBN
Paperback 979-8-89610-286-1
Hardcase 979-8-89699-347-6

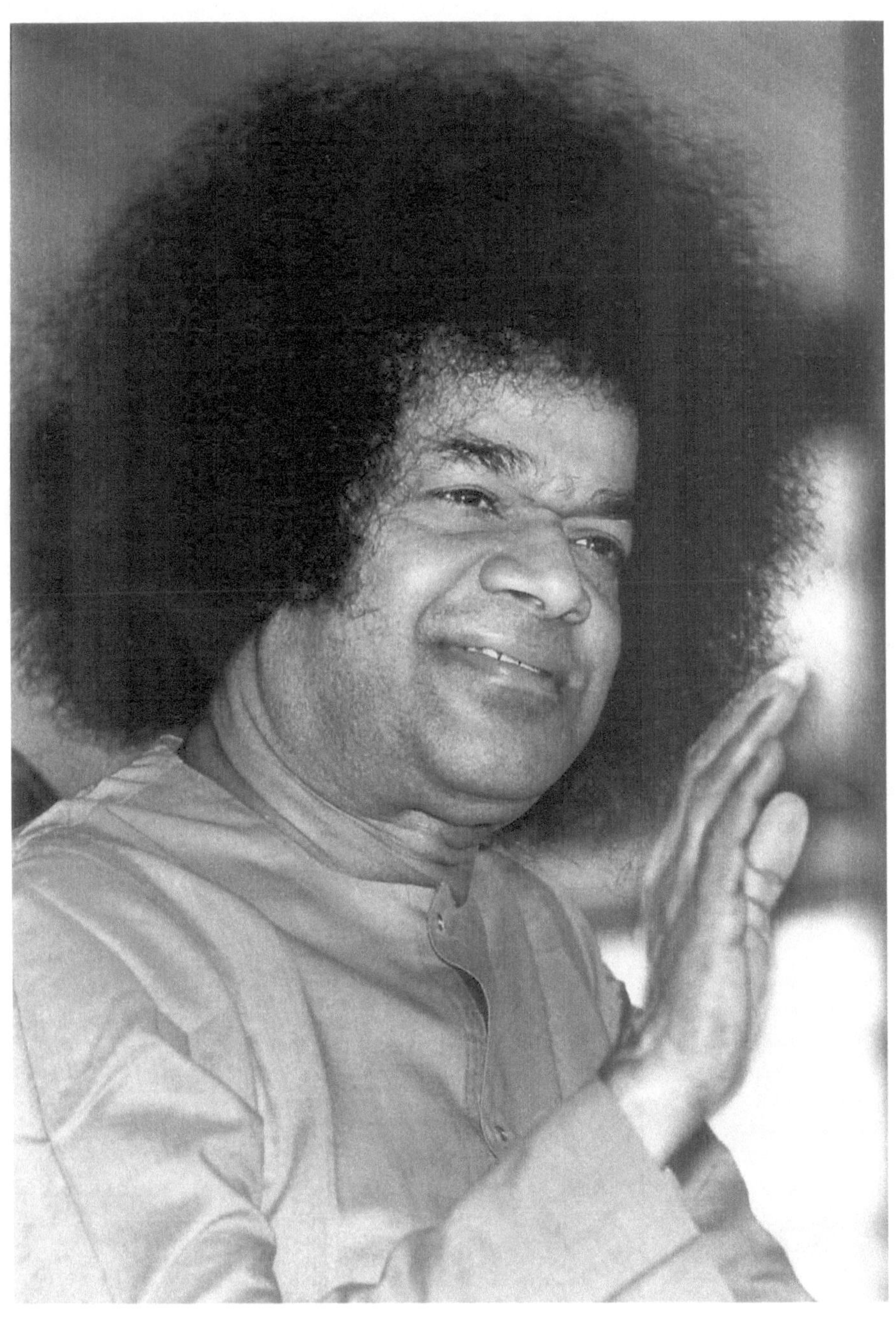

My humble Offering

The book 'Sai Ashtang Yoga' is
Dedicated at the Divine Lotus Feet
Of my beloved God and Guru
Bhagawan Sri Sathya Sai Baba

Contents

'Gratitude'

"You must show gratitude with humility and sincerity to whoever has done to you any good".

– Sri Satya Sai Baba

Acknowledgements

My humble Pranams, with love and gratitude at the Divine Lotus Feet of my Beloved God and Guru Sri Sathya Sai Baba, for inspiring me and making me an instrument in writing this book. Without His Grace, it would have been impossible for me to write this book.

I offer my heartfelt gratitude to my beloved parents who laid the foundation, on which this spiritual edifice is built.

I express special thanks to my editor Dr. Sue Evans for taking out time from her busy schedule for editing this book and for her insightful comments on the manuscript.

I am extremely grateful to Vinay and Sandhya (my brother & sister-in-law) for going through the final manuscript and for their valuable suggestions on it.

My thanks, love and gratitude to all my family members, without whose support it would not have been possible for me to complete this book, especially my little daughter (in-law), Shweta, both my sons Chetan & Siddharth and last but not least, love and thanks to my best friend, my husband, Deepak (official name Shailendra) who has been a great support in many ways.

My Pranams with love to Late Mr. Mahadevbhai Joshi who has unknowingly been a great support in increasing my knowledge by sharing valuable spiritual books.

Lastly, I am grateful to all who have supported me, knowingly or unknowingly, with their helpful suggestions and also helping me personally.

DR. KAVITA S. BHATT

'Discipline'

"Discipline is essential from the moment of waking to the time of going to sleep. It has to be a natural component of one's daily life in the discharge of one's duties".

– *Sri Satya Sai Baba*

Introduction

WHAT IS SAI ASTANG YOGA?

It is a way of life, based on **the teachings of Sri Sathya Sai Baba** which when practiced will lead to good physical and mental health, good relationships and finally leads to liberation.

In the prescribed study and practice of Yoga the 1st step is understanding and practicing the eight stages of Yoga. Yoga teaches us to live in balance and extinguish negative emotionalities. It teaches the balance of all things and balance **in** all things. **Moderation is the Key Word.**

"Sai Astanga Yoga" means – As this book is based on Sai's teachings, it starts with the word **"Sai". "Astang"** means 8 limbs or steps or stages, i.e. **Asta** means eight and **Anga** means limbs. "Yoga" means union or to join. Hence **"Sai Astang Yoga"** is a way of life, based on Sai's teachings which if practiced sincerely and regularly will lead us to union with the ultimate.

The practices mentioned in this book are not to make a person professional in Yogic studies, but for practical purposes. The practices explained here are simple and can be followed by people of all ages. Only a few important practices, especially in Asana, Mudra, Bandhas and Pranayama are delta-with, taking into consideration the hectic schedule and time constraints of day to day life.

The 8 essential stages in the study and practice of Yoga are:

1) **YAMA or Abstinence from or to keep away from:**
   b) **Shad Ripus or 6 enemies i.e.**
      Kama- Lust,
      Krodha – Anger,
      Lobha – Greed,
      Moha – Attachment,
      Madha – Pride,
      Matsar – Envy or Jealousy.
      By controlling our Desires we can keep away or abstain from Shad Ripus. Hence,
   c) **Ceiling on Desires:** Keeping desires under control or to place a ceiling on them. How to reduce desires? We will understand (explained in the following Chapters) how by not wasting food, money, time and energy, we can control desires.

2) **NIYAMA or Observance or to follow:**
   Sathya – Truthfulness,
   Dharma – Righteousness,
   Shanti – Peace,
   Prema – Love and
   Ahimsa – Non-violence.

3) **ASANAS: (The Classical Postures):**
   Asana means the position which is steady and comfortable by the practice of which we develop the ability to sit in one position without discomfort for a longer time, which is useful during meditation. Asanas help the body to become supple and flexible.

4) **PRANAYAM: (Breathing Techniques / Life force control)**
   Pranayam means regulation of breath or control of breath i.e. control of Prana or life-force. It is the sum total of all the forces in nature, latent forces in us and all around us. Heat, light, electricity and magnetism are all manifestations of Prana.

5) **PRATYAHAR: (Sense-Withdrawal / Mind Control):**
   Pratyahar or sense-withdrawal means 'Mastery of the senses'. When the mind detaches itself from the external objects, sense withdrawal occurs.

The sense organs which are normally extroverted are trained to become introverted and in-turned, sense withdrawal is attained.

6) **DHARANA:** means Concentration and Contemplation.
Concentration is a conscious effort to focus the mind on the object of concentration free of all distraction. When concentration becomes single-minded and the object of concentration is held by the mind itself; then it is contemplation.

7) **DHYANA:** means **Meditation.** When the focus of attention is maintained through dharana, unbound by time and space, it becomes Dhyana or meditation. Meditation is a process of treading the inward path to reach the destination of the Real Self.

8) **SAMADHI:** means Equipoise. 'Sama' means equal and 'Dhi' means Buddhi. Hence Samadhi means equal mindedness. Samadhi is the climax stage of meditation. It means complete absorption in the self.

The **first four** stages are called the **outer or gross steps** while the **last four** stages are called **the inner or subtle steps.**

Yama and Niyama are worked at together.

The Asanas and Pranayam are worked at together.

By Practice of Yama and Niyama:

1) The objective of the first four stages of Yoga is to cleanse the mental and physical body of physical and mental phlegm.

2) By following Yama and Niyama there is a change in our basic attitude. The study of these two steps will bring a drastic change in our intellectual understanding and thus bring a change in our thought pattern which in turn will bring a change in our attitude.

3) We become more positive (by the practice of Niyama) and cleansing of negativity (Shad Ripus) takes place; we learn to channelize and discipline our life.

4) We understand the deeper meaning of life and have a sense of self-satisfaction because by the practice of Yama and Niyama we start functioning from the conscious level (divine level) and not from the Ego level (personal level)

5) The cleaning of the mind is cleansing of the astral channels or Nadis. This cleansing takes place so that the life force can flow through astral channels activating greater self consciousness and greater balanced self conscious awareness within ourselves (Called "Nadi Sudhi" in our scriptures or one may say purification of the mind.)

6) All **Niyama** are **Divine qualities**. By following them we move more closer to divinity.

By Practice of Ceiling on Desires: By keeping control over the five essentialities of life viz. Food, money, time, energy and knowledge, we can achieve ceiling on desires, or control over our desires which is an essential factor for the practice of Yama and Niyama.

By Practice of Asana and Pranayama:

1) It becomes easy to control thought. Breath is connected with thought. For example, when we experience fear our breathing becomes faster. Hence if we control breath, we can control thought.

2) Body and mind become supple and flexible and relaxed. Asana make the body supple and pranayama or breath controls and relaxes the mind.

3) The nervous system in the physical body and the astral channels in the astral body get cleansed so that life force or Prana can flow smoothly and activate greater self consciousness, self awareness and greater balance within ourselves.

4) Nerves in our physical body are the only part of the body that **never re-generate** during our life time.

5) The astral channels or Nadis are super premental channels by which consciousness reaches out into infinity and contact can be made with the spiritual life forces by Pranic Energy flowing through our astral channels.

By practicing Yama-Niyama, Asana and Pranayama our body and mind gets totally healed and becomes a perfect vehicle for further spiritual progress.

THE FOUR INNER STAGES OR STEPS:

PRATYLAHAR or Sense Withdrawal is a yogic technique by which we take the naturally extroverted and outgoing forces of the sense organs and cause them to become introverted. This is done by drawing the senses away from their respective objects.

It also means, 'mastery over senses'. When mind detaches itself from the external objects sense withdrawal occurs. For example, sometimes we are in our own world, thinking, and even though a person walks in front of us we do not see him) The key word is **detachment – not detachment from the objects but DETACHMENT FROM REACTIONS to these objects.**

DHARANA or Concentration and Contemplation. As Sense withdrawal is mastered, concentration begins, which leads to Contemplation and when finally these two are mastered **Meditation** or **DHYANA** commences, which ultimately leads to **SAMADHI or Equipoise.**

The timing of beginning and ending of each stage cannot be said or measured. These separate movements occur simultaneously with eminent speed when one sits for practicing the inward path. It is for purpose of explanation that we break down yoga into parts.

CONCLUSION:

Yama and Niyam clean the mind states, the subtler astral channels.

Asanas and Pranayam tend to cleanse the physical and astral channels. The two working together cleanse the total vehicle of our mind and body, so that the energies can flow through the astral channels to the opposite end reaching into the causal plane of God-Consciousness. These outer stages reach their perfection in the 4th stage called Pranayama which controls the Pranic life force through breathing procedures.

After practicing Yama, Niyam, Asanas and Pranayam, our physiological or Physical activities get well harmonized and come under control. The next thing to follow is to fill the gap between the body and mind through psychosomatic or psychological training with a view to controlling the external and internal senses which affect the equanimity and peace of mind.

The thinking mind or the Ego is the perceiver and the thinking mind or Ego is the enjoyer. Mind or Ego is the only factor which attaches in Bandhan or Bondage and detaches in Moksha or Liberation.

Mind is in bondage because of **Trishna (greed)**, **Vasana or Upabhog (Lust)**, **Icehha (desire)** and **Maheccha (big desires-** big desires like planning for future) All greed and desires are because of Senses.

HENCE CEILING ON DESIRES.

In the following eight Chapters, we will explore in turn each of the eight steps of 'Sai Astang Yoga'. We will start with 'Yama' or abstinence from Shad Ripus or 6 enemies - the root causes of desire.

SAI RAM

Chapter 1
Yama or Abstinences

In this Chapter, we will consider two aspects of Yama, controlling our desires (Ceiling on desires) and abstinence from the six enemies that result from uncontrolled desires.

The family that holds us captive

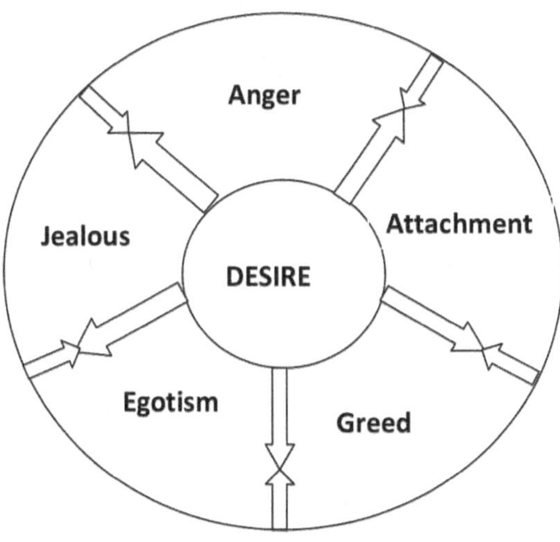

FAMILY NAMED SELFISHNESS

First step in developing our character is to liberate ourselves from the clutches of a family that holds us in slavery. It is a family of mother and her five children. Mother's name is **Desire**. When we desire something intensely and do not get it, the twins **Anger and Jealousy** are born. On the other hand, if we do get it the third child arrives, named **Attachment**. As our attachment grows, and we want more of the same, the fourth child is born, named **Greed.** As our Greed gets satiated, the youngest one arrives, named **Egotism.**

My beloved God and Guru **Sri Sathya Sai Baba's advice** is to put the mother to sleep and He says, "I guarantee that the children will vacate the house named X, Y or Z". This advice is reflected in the famous equation below:

$$\text{Happiness} = \frac{\text{Number of desires fulfilled}}{\text{Number of desires entertained}}$$

The equation for happiness suggests that if we have the will power to control our desires and keep them limited then our happiness quotient goes up. The lesser the denominator – the number of desires entertained – the higher will be our peace of mind and happiness.

(Source: Education in Human Values – a course book for training of Masters)

A SMALL STORY:

How desire leads to Shad Ripus.

*A young boy, Avinash, was very poor but very ambitious and wanted to be rich,.(**Desire**). He was working for a small private firm and worked very hard. He was living in a one room kitchen flat. He studied further and got a comparatively better job. He desired an airline job with the influence of his friend.*

*He could not get an airline job hence he was frustrated, **angry and jealous.***

*After struggling for some time, he got a job in a bank with a substantial rise in his salary. Now he purchased a one bed- room, hall, kitchen flat. He was respected by all and was happy. He further studied and completed his M.B.A. He became more **attached (Moha)** to money. He now wanted to earn more money. Good luck prevailed and he got a job in a foreign bank. He purchased a three bed room hall kitchen flat. Once there is attachment for money it grows and becomes **Greed.** He became **proud and Egoistic.** He forgot his old days and started treating his juniors very rudely. Because of Greed he fell prey to taking bribes and was caught red- handed by the management and lost his job.*

*This story shows how **Desire** leads to **Shad Ripus** and if we fall prey to them, how we lose our mental peace, which further leads to frustration and depression etc.*

YAMA OR ABSTINENCES

(To Keep Away from)
Desires and Shad Ripus or 6 Enemies

1) KAMA - Lust

2) KHRODHA - Anger

3) LOBHA - Greed

4) MOHA - Attachment

5) MADH - Pride (boosts Ego)

6) MATSAR - Envy or Jealousy

YAMA:

1

Kama or Lust: The First Shad Ripu

To abstain from Kama or lust, we must follow celibacy or Brahmacharya.

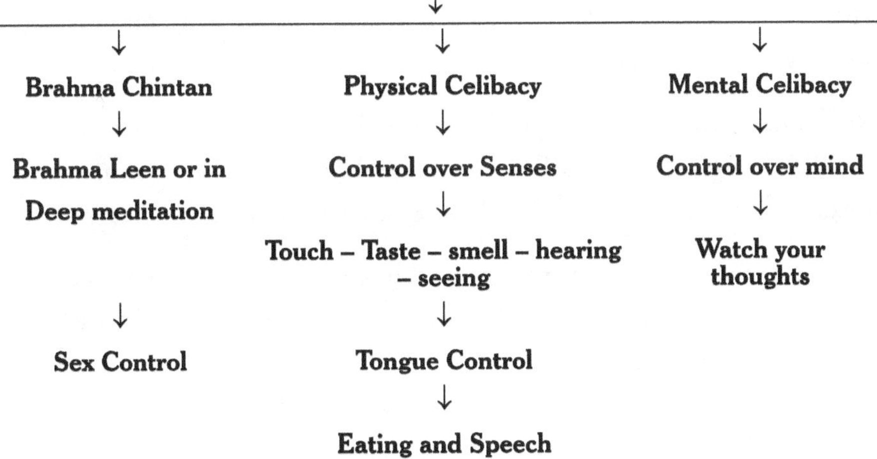

Brahmacharya: 3 Steps:

1) Spiritual Level: One who does Brahma chintan or meditates on Brahman is a Brahmachari

2) At Physical Level: Keeping away from Sensual or Sense attraction or Sense Control, Sex Control – Celibacy.

3) At Mental Level: Controlling the mind, not being judgmental, gossiping and criticism.

1) **Spiritual Level:** Brahma chintan means, one who is all the time thinking of or is (stith) fixed in Brahman or in deep meditation.

2) **At Physical Level: Control over senses – Touch- i.e. Sex Control, Taste – i.e. Tongue Control in eating and speech, smelling, hearing and seeing.**

Touch – i.e. Sex Control: Sex is one of the facets or aspects of life and the absolute or God which wishes to multiply. So sex is a must for Grahasta. First comes procreation and hence sex should be used with discrimination.

1) Pajan- Body union
2) Udatikaran- to go to higher level of consciousness – emotionally, intellectually and sentimentally.

In the actual process of body union the mental state is such that the mind is elevated to the highest emotional, intellectual and sentimental level. In this process for some point it becomes one with God i.e. one with the Universal Mind (God's Mind). Thus when there is a total union of body, mind and soul then there can be a new creation.

One more important point to be noted here is that when there is total union, the Muladhara Chakra or the Root charkra which is situated between the genital organ and the anus is also activated. Now this activation has two aspects:

1) when there are good and pure thoughts during the act, there are chances that the Kundalini Shakti is activated which is dormant at the Muladhara.
2) If there are bad or impure thoughts then they give the negative effect to the body and mind. So here everything depends on the mind.

Taste – i.e. Tongue Control: The aspirant should have complete control over his tongue in eating as well as speech. **Mauna or observing silence** gives a very important role to Tongue control as well as thought control. Similarly all other senses like **seeing, hearing and smelling also play an important role in KAMA, which also means UNNECESSARY DESIRES. Hence sense control gives control over DESIRES.**

At Mental Level: Control over the mind – watching the thoughts.

When we start watching our thoughts we stop being JUDGEMENTAL, we also stop gossiping and criticism.

> ## *A SMALL STORY:*
>
> *A man named Pankaj was very fond of cars and one day he purchased a new expensive car. He had learnt driving at the driving school. One day he decided to go round the town alone without the trainer. He started the car and drove it slowly for sometime and then gained speed. Soon he lost control of the car and the car went zig zag and ultimately dashed a tree and stopped.*
>
> *A friend Vinod, who was passing by, saw his condition and came to help him. He asked him in surprise, "Why are you driving the car when you don't know how to drive? And that too such an expensive car!"*
>
> *Pankaj replied "Do you mean to say I don't know to drive? Of course I know how to drive; I just don't know how to stop!"*

Most of the time we are in a similar situation, like Pankaj, who did not know how to stop the car but only knew how to start and move it ahead. He was not driving the car but the car was driving him! Similarly, most of us have no control over our mind; our mind controls us. Ultimately mind is nothing but a bundle of thoughts so if there is no clarity in our thinking, it only shows that we have too many contradicting thoughts crowding in our mind.

Being **JUDGEMENTAL** means passing comments about others thinking that one knows everything about others. **Gossiping** means unnecessarily talking about others and **Criticism** means finding faults with others. In being JUDGEMENTAL, gossiping and criticizing others the mind is involved in unnecessary negative thinking because of which the EGO is boosted.

Therefore my Guru and God **Sri Sathya Sai Baba** always say that '**Forget the good you have done to others and forget the harm that others have done to you**'. We all have our own nature, which is a mix of positive virtues and negative qualities. So understanding this we must always see the good in others and understand our own negative qualities and try to eliminate them. This is true mental celibacy.

A SMALL STORY:

Once two well-built and handsome celibates/yogi's were chit-chatting and walking towards a river. On the bank of the river they saw a beautiful young girl confused as to how to cross the river. Both of them enquired as to what the problem was. The girl explained her dilemma. One of the Yogis offered to carry the girl in his arms and cross the river. Thus both the celibates walked into the deep waters, one carrying the girl in his arms. When they reached the opposite bank, the girl stepped down, thanked the yogi and walked her way.

These two celibates walked to their ashram.

The one who saw his friend carrying the girl in his arms was uneasy and could not sleep for entire night. Next day, early in the morning he went to his friend and asked him, 'Don't you think it was against Bramhacharya or celibacy to touch a young and beautiful girl?'

The friend then replied, 'I was just helping the girl to cross the river and forgot all about her as soon as she stepped down, but you have been carrying her the entire night in your head. Is this not against Bramhacharya or celibacy?'

We are normal Human being and there is every chance that once in a while, we may get off track in our practices. Here one important thing to be noted, that no **guilt feeling should be allowed to set in our mind,** for guilt creates a lot of physical and mental pain. Make a note of the mistake and see that you don't repeat it next time. Hence learn to forgive your-self.

Now let us understand the second shad ripu – Krodha or anger.

SAI RAM

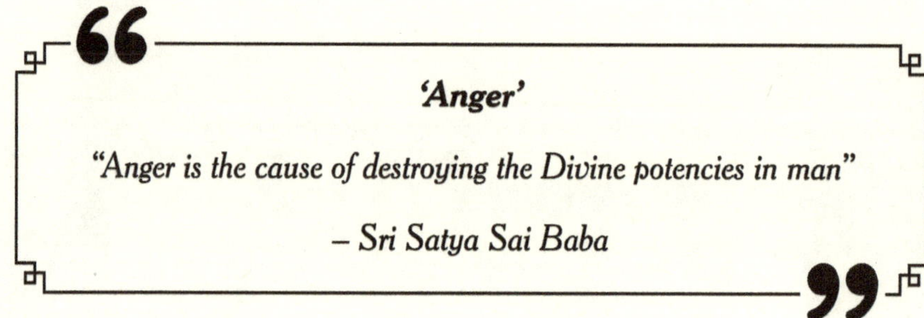
'Anger'
"Anger is the cause of destroying the Divine potencies in man"
– Sri Satya Sai Baba

2

Khrodh or Anger –
The Second Shad Ripu

KHRODHA OR ANGER

I) Causes of Anger

Internal

1) Non fulfillment of desire.

2) Short tempered

3) Ego

4) Fear

External

1) Instigation

2) Injustice

3) Failure

4) Non fulfillment of command or wish.

5) Deprivation of something.

II) Types of Anger

1) Impulsive

2) Mounting

3) False Anger

III) Symptoms

1) Fast and unrhythmic breathing

2) Increase in body temperature

3) Mental faculty does not function Properly.

IV) Why anger is bad

1) High body temperature and B.P.

2) Loss of mental equilibrium.

3) Spoils relationships.

4) Converts beauty into beast.

5) Heavy drain of Energy

6) Labeled as 'Bad Tempered'

V) Control of Anger

1) Namasmarana

2) Drink a glass of water

3) Change of place

4) Lie down

5) View your face in the mirror

6) Hold the middle finger of either hand.

VI) How to avoid anger

1) Use of discrimination power

2) Give up Ego

3) Develop Love (Ekatma Bhava)

4) Forbearance –develop tolerance

5) Ceiling on Desires

KHRODHA OR ANGER:

Kama, Krodha, Lobha, Moha, Madha, Macchar are our 6 enemies.

Anger is the worst among all. Swami says anger turns a man into drunken brute.

I) Causes of Anger:

Internal Causes:

1) **Non fulfillment of Desire:-** When our desires are not fulfilled we get angry. For example, you have planned to go for a movie with a friend and you are already late. The door bell rings and also the phone rings and the person on the other side of the line keeps on talking, even if you do not show interest in talking to him since you will miss the beginning of the movie. And this results in anger.

2) **Short tempered:-** It is the nature of man. Some people are by nature short tempered and so they get angry fast and sometimes without valid reason. Most of the time people who are impatient also get angry fast because things do not happen as per their time.

3) **Ego:-** Identifying self with the body and mind is Ego. So when injustice is done to body or mind (mental hurt) causes anger.

> ### *A STORY:*
>
> *Alexander had conquered half the world and had also invaded India many times. At one such time after the invasion he reported back to Greece. In those days too everyone was aware of the Spiritual heritage of India and so, he was told by the ministers and the people of Greece to bring along a sage from India along with the wealth of India. Alexander went to the Himalayas to find the sage. In one of the caves he comes across a sage in a deep meditational trance. Alexander was full of ego of his victory and in anger he shouted at the sage to wake up. The sage slowly opened his eyes and seeing Alexander, told him politely to sit.*
>
> *The sage enquired, "Who are you? And what do you want?" Alexander replied - "I am the King of Kings. I want you to come with me to Greece."*
>
> *The sage replied, "You don't seem to look like the king but a slave."*
>
> *Alexander was shocked and asked for justification. The sage said, "My anger is my slave and I have full control over it; whereas you get angry and so you are a slave of slaves." Alexander was shocked to hear this statement and also stunned to see the self confidence and body language of the sage.*

So when we become egoistic and get angry, we only display our own low self esteem.

4) **Fear:-** Fear also causes anger. The fear of being exposed or fear because we are hiding something often leads to anger. We start shouting and abusing/ accusing in order to dodge the issue. Swami says… Sometimes the cloud of envy and hatred comes to darken relationship. This is primalarily due to fear, fear that causes anger.

External Causes:

1) **Instigation:-** When someone instigates us or provokes us the natural out -come is anger.

2) **Injustice:-** Injustice to self and also injustice to others leads to anger. Man's innate nature is Dharma – Justice therefore we cannot see or bear injustice, and when we do, we get angry.

3) **Failure:-** When we fail to do something we get angry. Sometimes our failure to do something causes anger to come out on others. For example: We are late to start from our house so we blame the traffic, the signal and all things under the sun cursing them for delaying us in reaching our destination. It is so because we always think that the fault lies there, we do not realize that the fault lies here.

4) **Non fulfillment of command or wish:-** When we are in a position to command and our order is not carried out we get angry. For example, we command our assistant to complete the work and then go home, but the assistant does not obey us then we get angry.

   OR

   When we wish for something from our seniors, elders or employer and when our wish is not granted we get angry. For example, we apply for leave from office to attend a function and if it is not granted then we get angry because our wish to attend the function is not fulfilled.

5) **Deprivation of something:-** When we are deprived of something which we want or we deserve, we get angry especially when we think that we deserve it for example, Promotion, or a child feels deprived when it sees the toy in another child's hand.

ii) Types of Anger:

1) **Impulsive:-** When we react impulsively i.e. without deep thinking we get angry. There is a scientific reason behind it. When we react impulsively/ instantly we allow the HYPO-THALAMUS to handle the problem. The THALAMUS is an egg-sized bunch of nerve cells just below the brains cerebellum and is considered the **hot- headed seat of emotion.**

Instead if we wait a few seconds before blowing up, by responding, we automatically send our emotions to the cooling front office of the brain or the cerebellum, which is likely to process our anger in a rational manner. We often see that the outcome of the actions due to impulsiveness is bad. We realize this when it is too late and then we think if we had not behaved in this manner this would not have happened. Hence always **respond** do not **react.**

2) **MOUNTING:** leads to **outburst.** Someone goes on instigating us and we do not answer back because we have decided to remain calm. But when our tolerance level is reached, everything comes out in an outburst.

3) **FALSE ANGER:** Is there anything like false anger? Yes, there is. Sometimes mother gets angry at her child and scolds or even beats him/her but the anger directed towards the child is not real. The mother never likes to scold her child. She is weeping from inside but for the good of her child she has to be firm.

iii) Symptoms:

1) Fast and unrythmic breathing
2) Body temperature goes up.
3) Mental faculties do not function normally.

iv) Why is Anger Bad?

1) **Raises body temperature and Blood Pressure:-** It spoils health. Anger weakens the body: 3 months of energy drains with one strong bout of anger. It impairs the digestive system and chases man fast into old age. Fever and sprains are caused by suppressed anger.

2) **Lose of equilibrium:-** Anger leads to imbalance of mind, faulty decision and wrong action. Swami says – Anger is the stickiest dirt. When we get angry, we forget mother, father and teacher, we lose all discrimination in the excitement for example. Even Hanuman set fire to the whole Lanka when he was inceased by the Rakshasas who set fire to the tip of his tail.

He lost sight of the fact that Sita was in the Ashoka Van. It was only when he had exulted in achievement for a little while that he remembered it and then he started condemning himself for his anger.

3) **Spoils relationship:** What keeps two people together or families together is LOVE. Love is the energy that binds our relationships. But when we get angry we forget everything. You abuse another and he does the same, and temper rises, heat is generated and lasting injury is done. Five minutes of anger damages the relationship for five generations.

4) **Anger converts Beauty into Beast:-** When we get angry, we act as if we are possessed by an evil spirit, our face becomes ugly and frightful. As a matter of fact, like the red bulb winking when danger is approaching the eyes and face become red as a warning.

5) Anger is a **heavy drain on our energy** and a big enemy. Swami says.... One attack of anger exhausts 3 months of health and efficiency e.g. Before encountering Jarasandha in open battle Krishna enraged him nine times; time after time getting nearly caught and escaping from his hold; these bouts of rage so weakened him that, when the final bout took place, he could be easily over- powered.

6) You are labeled as "BAD TEMPERED".

v) Control of Anger:

1) **Namasmarana:** Chanting of God's name always gives us peace of mind.

   Like Krishna danced with his tender feet on the hood of Kali Nag and removed the poison from his five fangs, let the sweet name of the lord dance on our tongue and he will remove the poison from our five enemies. With that anger will also go away.

2) **Drink a glass of water** at room temperature. It will reduce the temperature of the boiling blood by diluting the impact of toxic chemicals and secretions created in the body due to anger. E.g. once a lady was quarrelling too much while standing in the line for filling water. A lot of heated exchange of words took place and the fight took a very violent turn. The lady, still in a fit of fury came home and immediately

fed her infant. The child died immediately. This was due to the toxic chemicals anger secreted in her body, got mixed with the milk, with the result the child died.

3) **Change of Place:** Physically get away from the scene of anger to get out of negative, harmful vibrations.

4) **Lie down:** (Anger will subside) Anger travels in a vertical plane and never in a horizontal plane. If we are lying down and someone says something bad to us, we immediately get up and answer back. We rarely quarrel lying down. Also we see that when some old person in our house gets angry, others tell them to lie down for a while.

5) **Watch the face** in the mirror. One glance at yourself will make anger vanish.

6) **Hold the middle finger of either hand** to control anger. Anger is such a negative force that it separates the soul from the body because it creates such an intense, destabilizing energy within which badly affects the functioning of the liver, gall bladder and the pancreas. Holding of the middle finger harmonizes the liver and gall bladder, which helps to control the anger.

vi) How to Avoid Anger?

1) **Use of discrimination power:** Do not allow the THALAMUS to handle the situation. Let our intellect make the decision instead of our mind. Because the mind is like a receiving clerk in the office, while intellect is the officer-in-charge who makes the decisions.

2) **Give up Ego:** Remember the faults we see in others are faults within us.

3) **Develop Love:** Ekatma Bhav. See God in every one. "Brotherhood of man and Fatherhood of God." We are sparks of the same Divine.

4) **Forbearance: (Sahana or tolerance):** Swami says…. We cannot destroy anger by anger. Anger can be subdued only by forbearance….. Sweet tolerance. Remember, "Anger is the chief enemy of Sadhana". To get angry is but the effort of a moment; but to get peace, to become unaffected by the ups and downs of life is the result of years of training in Vedanta.

5) **Ceiling on Desires:** We cannot get everything in life; all our experience of life shows us that. Hence Swami says, always be AWARE of the desires, whether it is a NEED or GREED and select according.

After understanding the two Shad Ripus namely Kama or lust and Krodha or anger we move on to the third shad ripu, Lobha or greed.

SAI RAM

3

Lobha or Greed – The Third Shad Ripu

LOBHA OR GREED

↓(1)	↓(2)	↓(3)
Inner wealth or well-being	The illogical monkey mind	Craving
↓	↓	

(1)		(2)		
↓(a)	↓(b)	↓(a)	↓(b)	↓(c)
The quality of life not quantity of wealth.	Need or Greed Diff. between craving and enjoyment	Horizontal and Vertical thinking	The Brain Nurounic layer, enjoying things mentally	Living in the not Present, within boundary.

I) LAKSHMI-THE GODDESS OF INNER WEALTH AND WELL-BEING

a) The quality of life and not the quantity of wealth.

b) Need or Greed – Difference between craving for things and enjoying them.

A SMALL STORY FROM THE GREAT HINDU EPIC, THE MAHABHARARTA:

A great king named Yayati was living comfortably, enjoying his life. He lived for 100 Years, and it was time for him to exit from the world. Yama, the God of death came to take him. On seeing Yama the King was shocked and started pleading, "Why have you come so suddenly without any notice. I still have to live my life for some more time, so please give me some more time to live!"

Yama said that he could not go against the laws of nature and hence it was not possible to give him extension of his destined span of life.

Yayati begged and pleaded for some more time.

So Yama gave him one option saying that if one of his sons could give their life for him than he could get extension.

Yayati was happy, called one of his sons and requested him to give some part of his life so that he could survive. The son loved his father, gave up the remaining years of his life and died instantly. Thus Yayati was granted another 100 years by Yama.

At the end of this period Yama again visited Yayati. This time again the King begged and pleaded for further extension of his life span. This time too one of his sons gave up his life for his father and Yayati got a lease of 100 years once again.

Now as Yayati was busy enjoying his life and was unaware of the passage of time, Yama came back to take him.

As Yayati started pleading again, Yama looked compassionately at the King and said "Oh! Great King, Do you think you can put off a fire by pouring oil into it? Do you think you can satisfy and fulfill all your endless desires by living them out more and more?"

At this moment Yayati realized the truth in his statement and followed Yama Immediately to the divine abode.

The Mahabharata explains that, on hearing Yama's statement Yayati experienced the riches of the inner being that is **Lakshmi, (the Goddess of wealth)** which finally made him realize the truth and hence he followed Yama to the divine abode. Lakshmi symbolizes the richness of the inner world and enhances the quality of life.

Ia) The Quality of Life and Not the Quantity or Wealth

Rich and wealthy people would have led the best quality of life, if and only if money, wealth and possession could do that. Hence the quantity of wealth and riches does not mean best quality of life. It is a fact that we all need money to lead a reasonably comfortable life but even if we have all the wealth in the world, we may still be dissatisfied and discontented. There can be no fulfillment even though one has enough wealth. One thing we are not aware of is the deep-rooted need within us, which is beyond material wealth and possession, which tells us that there is a purpose of our life which is beyond this material success. Because we are so engrossed in the outside world, we are not aware of the inner feeling of discontent, and suffer because of it.

When we fail in our attempt to achieve something, we have the hope that the next time, we will be able to achieve success and there is this hope that keeps us going in life. But if we fail to achieve then there is depression and frustration which further detariots the quality of life. However, if we have already achieved everything and we are still not satisfied it is said to be **MOHA OR GREED**. Then there is nothing that gives us satisfaction through the material world.

For Example, when we are young; we yearn to settle in America, thinking that life there will be good. When we get there, we start working; buy a good house, thinking we will be happy after that. Once we get the house, we think that after marriage, life will be good. After marriage, we start feeling that when we have children, they will give us happiness. After having children, we start worrying about them and imagine that when they grow up and settle down we will finally be able to retire with money, be free from worries, and enjoy life.

However, by the time we retire, the mental set-up we have created to continuously run behind ' more and more' becomes a habit. We forget the art of enjoying life. Relaxation is only a word for us, not an experience. Naturally, we have lost sensitivity to life, the quality of enjoying life. It is like selling your eyes to purchase a beautiful painting; selling your sleep to buy a bed; selling your life to purchase a house.

When the ocean of milk (the mind) was churned by the devas (Gods) and rakshasas (demons) using the **Meru** mountain as a fulcrum and the giant serpent **Adi Sesha** as a rope to churn, from deep inside the ocean, **Lakshmi**, the Goddess of wealth emerged. This is just a metaphorical representation: When the mountain of pure awareness churns the ocean of milk, that is the mind, of its good and bad qualities it raises the quality of our lives in the form of Lakshmi.

Ib) Need or Greed

Difference Between Craving for Things and Enjoying Them

Most of us think that we crave for things because we enjoy them. No! If we are sensitive, our consciousness expands and we will only enjoy and never crave. The word enjoy means to enjoy what is there as reality, what is there in front of us at the given moment. For example, if I am staying in a one bed room, hall and kitchen flat and I am comfortable and happy with it, I will not crave for a three bed room, hall and kitchen flat. Just observe, we think of the three bed room flat only if we are not happy and satisfied with the one bed room flat. The thought of the three bed room, hall and kitchen flat will not surface in our range of consciousness if we are happy with our one bed room, hall and kitchen flat.

If we do not have the mindset to be happy and satisfied in the one bed room flat, be clear, we will not have the mindset to enjoy the three bed rooms flat either. The problem is not with the flats but with the mind.

So clearly understand, whether what you **WANT** is a **NEED OR GREED.**

A SMALL STORY:

Near a village, on the road- side, there was a big tree, but it had small leaves. Looking around, and seeing trees with large leaves, our tree was always unhappy. It craved for large size leaves. Seeing it sad, God granted its wish!

However, the large leaves attracted the villagers. They plucked them all for use as wrappers and for keeping eatables. The tree looked bare, and soon became sad once again. Use of its leaves for such purpose also made it very angry. It once again prayed fervently for a change; it wished for more valuable leaves, like gold. Now, this wish was also granted!

The villagers saw the glittering golden leaves, and plucked them all. They all became rich, therefore it prayed for leaves of glass with sharp edges which people would dare not pluck. Now no one could touch them.

It so happened that one day, the wind was very strong, and the tree started swaying on all sides. The glass leaves broke, and wounded the tree in many places. The tree was in acute pain, and cried in vain. It then realized that it is better to be content with what one has got, than desire for worldly attractions. Contentment brings happiness. Desires are the cause of dissatisfaction.

It repented, and prayed for its original size leaves. That wish too, God granted!

II) THE ILLOGICAL MIND – THE MAD MONKEY

a) **Horizontal and Vertical direction of thinking.**

b) **Brain Nurounic Layer – enjoying things mentally**

c) **Living in the Present.**

If we are aware we will realize that the mind is a most illogical instrument. When we watch our thoughts and write them, we will understand how illogical our mind is. It is as if we are running a mental asylum inside our heads! At one moment we think of our office and immediately for no reason, in the next moment we think about our home and even without our realizing, we think about our children. In actuality there is no connection, or no logic in the way our mind jumps from one thought to another. The association between thoughts is highly illogical.

And we have entrusted our whole lives to this mind of ours. Swami says that our mind is like a mad monkey that just jumps madly with no control over itself. The mind is not under our control; we are under *its* control.

When we analyze clearly, what is truth and eternal and what is untruth and ephemeral, from this intelligent analysis will arise our increased quality of life. When there is a feeling of satisfaction and contentment, we may say that we have acquired **Lakshmi**. The word Lakshmi stands not only for outer material wealth and prosperity but also the inner contentment, the inner richness which is the **quality of life or Being itself.**

IIa) Horizontal and Vertical Directions or Lines of Thinking

If we will observe our thinking pattern, we will notice that our thoughts move in a horizontal dimension i.e. What next? What next? As long as we are traveling on this horizontal plane, it is either Greed (endless desires) or Fear which is the driving force of our life and we keep on running after it till the end of our life.

All our thoughts, words and deeds are employed in satisfying our Greed and therefore we fail to enjoy the beautiful things in life. We always try to see if there is any benefit for us in everything that we come across. To travel in a horizontal dimension is a never-ending process. Our life is then based on craving and this will never allow us to taste life. We are always in a hurry to acquire and travel from more to more in the horizontal direction which ultimately leads us to our grave. For example; to a certain level, people drink alcohol and then alcohol starts drinking them. There are people who crave to eat. To a certain level it gives satisfaction but when they go beyond limits, the food starts eating them. So can we say we are leading a quality of life or is it that we are moving towards a slow death?

When we start directing our thought patterns in the vertical direction then we open up to another dimension of existence to our life and being called the **Vertical dimension.**

When we stop craving for more and more, we start living fully enjoying what we have. This gives us an inner deep satisfaction because we start living the reality. This deep satisfaction and contentment opens up a whole new dimension of life, and our enjoyment of what is already there increases.

Iib) Brain Nurounic Layer – Enjoying Things Mentally

Research had been conducted by the Psychologist in which it was discovered that if our mind is trained towards a philosophy of wanting 'more and more' or craving, then a new Brain Nurounic layer opens up where one starts enjoying mentally but not physically. This brain Nurounic layer stores all our imaginations and fantasies which we mentally enjoy, and not of the things we really possess. Without having them we just mentally enjoy them, that is all. For example, if one is staying in a rented house, the Brain Nurounic layer will be enjoying an apartment. When one goes to stay in the apartment, the Nurounic layer will already be staying in a bungalow! In this way one continuously **escapes reality.**

In our day-to-day life, we are unaware that we are continuously functioning in the Brain Nurounic layer. As we live in society, we have to follow certain norms or disciplines pertaining to society. There are many things we would want to do but because society does not permit it, we are unable to do it. For example, if we feel like dancing or wearing a particular fashioned dress in a public place, and we cannot, since society does not permit us to do so, what do we do? We satisfy ourselves vicariously by watching people dancing on or wearing a particular fashioned dress on television. Hence Swami says 'It is not

Television but TELEVISHUM'. It is nothing but **just mental enjoyment** and hence people get addicted to seeing television.

There can be an end to the physical enjoyment, when we get tired but there is no end to mental enjoyment as we keep on visualizing and we will never get tired! Is there any end to this mental enjoyment? No, there is no end to it. Therefore it is very dangerous.

When we continue to mentally enjoy, two things happen; firstly, we accumulate more and more fantasies from what we see. Secondly, we never get complete satisfaction and fulfillment through it.

Iic) Living in the Present – Living Within Our Limits

If we are aware, we will observe that our mind never stays where our body stays i.e. our mind is never present, wherever we are. It just keeps on wandering here and there. This is the life style of wanting more and more. Our mind makes us run all the time without even knowing what we are running for. Therefore drop the idea of greed or 'more and more'. Once we do this you will start living in the Present, in the Now.

For example, we get up in the morning and while we are brushing our teeth, we think about the train and how fast we can reach office. When we reach the office, we begin making plans for the evening, as some relatives are to visit our place, as to which restaurant we could visit. In the evening, we go to a restaurant, but once we are there, we are already tired and thinking about going home and resting. Similarly, on a Thursday at the office, we start thinking about how to spend the weekend. But when the weekend actually arrives, we start worrying about what work needs to be done in our office on Monday. On Monday, we are already thinking about the next weekend! By living in this fashion, we tire out very easily, because we function or do our physical actions in the present but our minds are thinking of the future, which creates a big gap between the body and the mind and this creates a lot of stress and tires us.

By the big gap that is created between the body and the mind; we postpone living in the present and constantly hope to live in the future. This postpones our enjoyment. The mind gets habituated to postponement and slowly this becomes our mental attitude. So **always remember**, what-ever you may acquire in terms of quantity, it is the **quality of life that gives it meaning.** We may have a beautiful house, but what is the use if we have no peace in it. So work to maintain mental peace and not to decorate it with unwanted furniture.

When we start living in the present, we start living in the now, there is a shift in our personal referral point which is called as a **cognitive shift.** When this happens there is intense awareness and our living is then centered in our being i.e. we start functioning from our conscious or divine level and we feel fulfilled. We are always in bliss. Life opens up a new dimension.

III) CRAVING

What is **craving?** Craving is a want which we do not have but we desperately want. So by just renouncing what we do not have, we can free ourselves from craving. Enjoy reality i.e. we are free to enjoy what we already have because it is ours and it will never disturb us. That which is not there, but troubles us as if it is there, is what is known as Maya or illusion. We are trying to continuously hold on to the illusion or maya of what we do not have through fantasizing and that is what craving is. So once we renounce what we do not have and enjoy only that which we already have, we are free from Maya or illusion.

A SMALL STORY

A man lived with his wife and their young son. They were very poor, and they came to the city in search of employment. Both the parents worked hard, but they could hardly make both ends meet. However, they took care of their son and sent him regularly to a nearby school.

> *The boy saw other children in the school and compared himself with them. He wore torn clothes, carried old and torn books, and walked barefoot. When returned back from school, he would complain to his parents about his condition, though the parents could afford nothing more than what they had already provided him.*
>
> *One day, the father and son were walking together towards the school, when the boy once again complained about his foot wear, "How can I go barefoot to school?' he said, "when all others wear shoes?" At that very moment, they both saw another boy, cheerfully trying to make his way towards the school. They noticed he had no feet.*
>
> ***"I cried that I had no shoes, till I saw him with no feet."*** *Be happy and contented with whatever you have.*

Drop our fantasies, our imagination about what we do not have.

CONCLUSION:

1) Quality of life improves which brings feel-good factor and well-being when we stop going after more. **Santoshi Nar Sada Sukhi** – One who is contented is always happy.

2) We are satisfied and start enjoying what-ever we have.

3) A good amount of control over our mind can be attained. There will be clarity of thought and illogical thinking will stop. We will be able to analyze our thought better, to understand what is temporary and what is permanent; what is right and what wrong, etc is. Our intellect will sharpen and we will feel fulfilled and satisfied with our life

4) Greed drives our thoughts, words and deeds. So without greed our thoughts, words and deeds are synchronized, and when thoughts, words and deeds are one, we function from the conscious or divine level.

5) We will be free from addiction. When psychologically we move out of the Brain Nurounic layer, the craving for wanting more will stop. Physical craving has an end but mental craving has no end.

6) Wanting more and more means living in future by fantasying for something or someone. By doing so we postpone our enjoyment when we constantly hope to live in the future. When we drop greed we start living in the present enjoying what is there in the present. When we live in the present we create a new mental setup or cognitive shift. We start living with awareness intensely.

7) Enjoying Reality and not fantasy i.e. Renounce what we do not have, and enjoy what we have. Hence give up craving and greed and have **Lakshmi** in our life or a better quality of live i.e. inner prosperity and richness.

God is not a manufacturer to mass-produce the same type of beings. He does not have a mould to turn out identical clay dolls. He is an artist who creates unique pieces of art in His creations. Each of us is as unique as every one of His unique creations. If we understand this, we will love ourselves and when we love ourselves we stop craving and asking for more and become free from **GREED.**

As we have already seen, greed and craving lead us to more and more desires, we now move to the next Shad Ripu – Moha or attachment

SAI RAM

'Attachment'

"*Do not get attached to worldly things and pursuits. Be in the world, but do not let the world be in you.*"

– *Sri Satya Sai Baba*

4

Moha – Attachment – The Fourth Shad Ripu

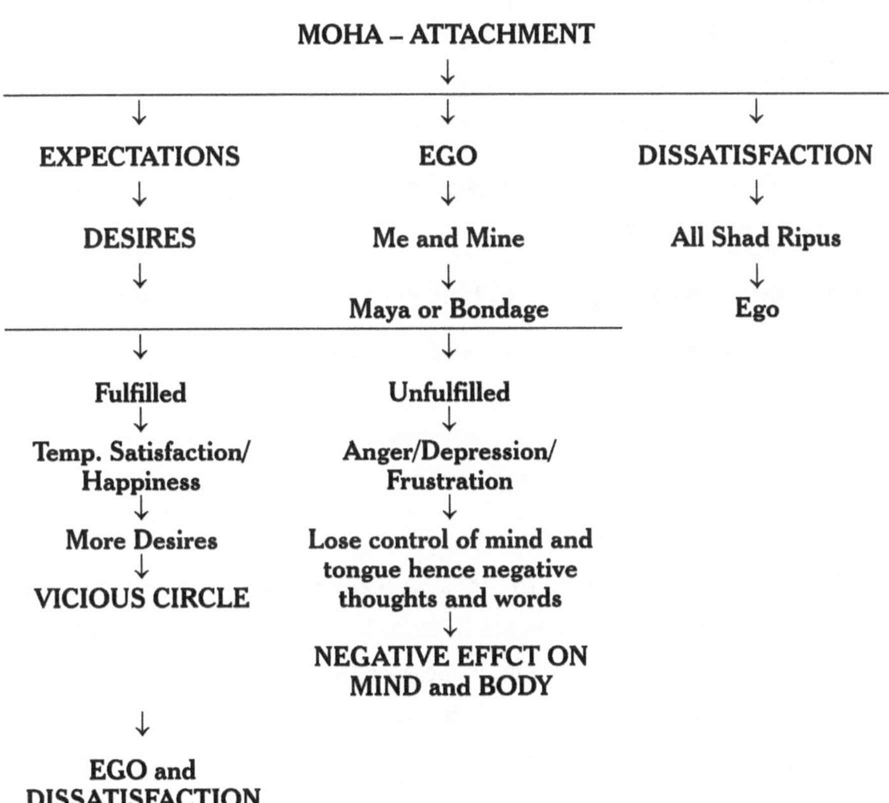

MOHA – MAYA:

Moha or attachment is always used with a suffix of Maya because Moha ultimately leads to Maya. **What is Maya? Maya is illusion. Another name for Maya is also Ego.** When the Ego or 'I' is not satisfied, it leads to **dissatisfaction** which further leads to Shad Ripus.

Moha or attachment is towards person, place or a thing.

Why do we get attached?

We get attached to a person, a place or a thing because

1) We feel comfortable with them.
2) We have a feel-good factor
3) We also have a feeling of security.
4) We are mentally not prepared for a change very easily.

Because of the above reasons and because we are a sensitive species with feelings and emotions we get attached very fast.

All attachments lead to EXPECTATIONS which further leads to DESIRES.

We are very much attached to our family members, relatives and friends and hence we expect from them, love, care, appreciation and acknowledgment in all that we think, say and do. These expectations are **small day-to-day desires.** These desires further lead to **bigger desires.**

There are 3 levels of desires:

1) **Physical Level:** the desire for physical pleasures and comforts, the desire to see beautiful things, desires to hear, desire to taste, smell and touch. The desire for sex. These are the basic pleasures because of the five senses. The desire to earn a lot of money and be rich.
2) **Mental Level:** The desire for name, fame, attention, love, care, appreciation etc.
3) **Spiritual Level:** The desire to be spiritual, the desire to have darshan (vision) of God and the desire for enlightenment, the desire to do selfless seva etc.

Analyze your desires deeply to see where you have a need and where it is merely greed. **If we analyze our mind or thoughts, our lifestyle, we can classify** our desires under these three categories. **IF OUR DESIRE IS COMING FROM THE HEART, IT IS NEED AND IF IT IS SOMEBODY ELSE'S, IT IS GREED.**

We have enough energy, power and capacity to fulfill our desires, but we do not have enough to fulfill the desires gathered from others. The fantasies that we pick up from the outer world are what disturb us. Reality in life never disturbs us;

For example, if we have a small car which serves our need or purpose, it is need (it is our own desire) and we want to have a bigger car because our friend has one (that is others' desires) then it is greed.

When our **desires are fulfilled**, there is **temporary satisfaction or happiness.** After sometime we want more, hence more desire and more attachment. The more desires are fulfilled the more we want and it is a **never ending vicious circle.** It is a dangerous whirlpool which ultimately leads to disaster.

When our **desires are not fulfilled, there is depression, frustration and anger;** we **lose control of our mind and tongue which gives rise to negative thoughts and words,** which further leads to **loss of energy and negative effects on mind and body creating diseases.**

A girl named Veena wanted to marry a boy Vinod of her choice, who was working with her in her office. Vinod was a sincere, hardworking and good-natured boy who belonged to a middle class family. The girl introduced Vinod to her parents. The parents had another boy in their mind from their own community who belonged to a rich and affluent family. There was a vast cultural difference between the two families, yet the parents insisted that Veena get married to the boy of their choice. This created a lot of discussion and heated arguments in the family, which further lead to abusing each other and there was disharmony in the family. Veena went into severe depression, the mother suffered from high B.P., and the father had a mild heart attack. This is how unfulfilled desires lead to anger, depression and frustration which cause mental and physical illness.

Another example is of our ministers and top class business persons. They are not ready to leave their chair or position which gives them name and fame and money.

Though Spiritual desires are good and positive desires, ultimately even those desires have to be dropped to just 'BE' i.e. TOTAL SURRENDER.

Thus all the desires fulfilled or unfulfilled lead to the BOOSTING OF THE EGO because of which we are in BONDAGE OR MAYA. Hence Swami (My divine God and Guru) teaches us to have CEILING ON DESIRES.

THE EGO:

What is Ego?

Ego is identification with the body and mind. It is the thought and feeling of 'I' in us. It is the reflection of the Real 'I' or divinity within us which is projected on the mirror of the mind. It is a fictitious entity which in actuality does not exist (ex. Our own image in the mirror).

The Ego too is the creation of God; it is His divine play or Leela for the creation to continue in duality as 'I' and 'You' and for the relationships to happen because of which the creation functions.

Understand that the 'I' i.e. ahamkar and 'MINE' i.e. mamakar keep us in maya i.e bondage.

'I' is the root of fear; 'mine' is the root of greed. The 'I' is the Ego and 'mine' is the sense of possession. We say this is mine that is mine, this is my car, this is my house, these are my relations, these are my friends etc. That is why the loss of the ego, the loss of 'I' seems so traumatic, so fearful.

The Ego being a false entity or reflection is always feeling insecure which creates fear.

Unless we throw ourselves into the utter insecurity of Existence, we will never experience real freedom, real bliss.

Bliss is choicelessness. If we try to make bliss a choice, it will be absent. If we can understand the purposelessness of life as a part of the grand Divine plan of Existence or the Divine Leela, we can reach that stage. That is to say, if we understand that we are not the doers and everything just happens as per His Divine plan and that we have absolutely no choice what so ever, we can reach a blissful state.

Ego or 'I' believes that there is purpose to life. It may be material, mental or spiritual. The more the purpose, the stronger our ego feels. If we drop all other purposes and still hold on to the purpose of enlightenment or self Realization, it is useless. Ultimately we have to give up the desire for self realization. Only when we understand and realize that life is totally purposeless and drop our ego will enlightenment or freedom happen to us.

One must understand that we are like water bubbles on the wave of the ocean. Similarly, there are other few bubbles holding on to the parent bubble which we name as father, son, husband, and wife. These bubbles are unaware that they may burst at any moment and hence collect sand particles thinking them to be jewels. Hence it is useless to think of possessing something and making thinking that it belongs to 'me'.

Our ego or the 'I' is stuck to the idea of purpose in life. The 'I' thinks that once it settles other social responsibilities it will take up the spiritual path. If we hold on to the idea of purpose in life, we start focusing on the goal of life and miss the path and also the joy of the path. Life will acquire meaning only when we are ready to accept that life is purposeless including physical, mental and spiritual objects.

The mind waits for something to happen all the time because it is either in the past or in the future. When we start calculating everything in terms of cost benefit, we reduce our spirit to matter.

BY DROPPING OUR EGO WE ARE IN BLISS and THE PURPOSE OF EXISTENCE IS BLISS: THAT IS ALL.

Dissatisfaction:

Why are we in search of happiness all the time? Because we are still not satisfied with what we have. When our desires are fulfilled we are still not satisfied and we want more and more. When the desires are not fulfilled then there is a great amount of dissatisfaction which leads to frustration, depression and ultimately to Shad Ripus. Dissatisfaction creates greed, anger, jealousy and pride i.e. it leads to becoming more **Egoistic.** This is how we are caught in a vicious cycle.

When we are caught in this vicious cycle of desires, we suffer from mental illness which further leads to physical diseases.

Attachment is the main cause for being possessive. Because of this we refer to everything that we possess as **"Me and Mine" i.e Ahamkar (Ego) and Mamakar** we tend to forget that nothing in this life is permanent, everything is temporary. This body, our relationships, our home and all the things we possess, everything is temporary. One day we all have to leave all this and leave for the heavenly abode. Inspite of knowing this we do not except this. **We live as if we will never die, and we die as if we have never lived.**

We have just seen how attachment leads to "me and mine" i.e. ego and possessiveness. Now let us understand what are pride i.e. Madh and jealousy i.e. Matshar

SAI RAM

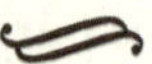

5 & 6

Madh – Pride (Ego) – The Fifth Shad Ripu

Matshar – Jealousy – The Sixth Shad Ripu

MADH – PRIDE OR EGO
↓
BORROWED DESIRES
↓
COMPARISION
↓
JEALOUSY

Even before we enter this planet earth, God makes provision for us by providing our parents to look after us, the total amount of food required by us, the house, the comforts and also the energy to fulfill all our desires. The capacity to enjoy all our desires and comforts is also given to us the moment we enter.

After coming down to this planet, we start enjoying life but we also see what others are enjoying. Now we want to enjoy our desires as well as the desires of others, so we start gathering desires from others. This is called **gathered desires. God has given us one life and also the energy to fulfill this one life's desires.** The problem starts when we start adding other's desires into our life because we do not have the capacity and energy to satisfy them. This results in greed and ultimately in stress

So we feel constantly that our time, energy and money are not sufficient; we feel deprived. Hence Swami teaches us to practice CEILING ON DESIRES i.e. right use of time, energy, food and money.

Mr. and Mrs. X went to a Mall to purchase a washing machine. On the way they met Mr. and Mrs. Y, who had been to purchase a coloured Television. Before meeting Mr. and Mrs. Y the X's were happy purchasing the washing machine. However now after meeting Y's they felt that they too should have colour T.V. Their life was perfectly alright without the television until then. Even the thought would not have crossed their minds. Now from where has the desire entered? From where did the disturbing thought about the television enter? Directly from the other person! This is exactly how we gather desires in every aspect of our lives, whether it is relationships or lifestyle or material things or anything.

Thus in our day-to-day life, we pick up lot of things from others and feel the pressure when we are not able to fulfill it.

So what is the deciding factor to understand if the desire is mine or a gathered one?

The answer is, if the desire gives us joy as it arises in us then it is our desire. There is a deep sense of satisfaction and fulfillment when we fulfill our desire. If it is a gathered desire; it will cause a sense of uneasiness. Even after we satisfy this desire it will leave behind a sense of guilt and discontentment. So check out if we feel tired or uneasy or if there is any disturbance in the mind, then there is something wrong somewhere.

Comparison:

With the intention of giving inspiration to a child he is compared with some other child. Even when there are two children in a family, the two are automatically compared in every situation, thus creating a sibling rivalry which is difficult to resolve later. Unknowingly this sows the seeds of comparison in us. And with comparison comes jealousy. Everything begins at home. So if comparison, naming and labeling of children as grades 1, 2, 3 etc is avoided then a lot of psychological problem faced by children today could be eradicated.

Different children have different aptitudes and inclinations. Some are good at visualizations and have natural inclination towards arts like painting, poetry, dancing etc.while some are good at verbalization; they become experts in the fields of logic and language. Some are good in other subjects. So when we grade children we generalize them and do not appreciate their respective abilities. In a way we are doing injustice to the innocent children.

Comparison, naturally leads to either **high self esteem** or **low self esteem.** So remember, when we compare we sow the seeds of misery. The element of jealousy is always present in comparison. We harbors the feeling of jealousy towards the other person when we have high self esteem. Unfortunately when there is low self esteem we get into a shell and suppress ourselves. There are chances of the **boosting of the Ego** when there is **high self esteem**. Such feelings are dangerous and the society does not support them and we may harbor mental violence in some form against society. So comparison should be avoided from a very young age so that we do not sow the seeds of jealousy in their tender hearts.

Thus comparison leads to jealousy and jealousy leads to mental violence; jealousy makes us pull other people down; we learn the method to stop the progress of others. The more we learn to compare, the more cunning and crooked we become. We keep on telling others 'How do we grow if we don't compare?' and thus continues the vicious cycle of comparison jealousy and violence.

Who is comparing and who is Jealous? It's none other than our EGO, which is nothing but just a reflection. One glimpse of this truth will remove jealousy and comparison from our system.

> ### *A STORY:*
>
> *In a village, there lived an old man with his 3 sons. He had a small business of his own. He was growing old and wanted to give his responsibilities to one of his sons who was capable of handling his business. So he decided to test them. He called all the three in a room and gave them rupees 3 each and told them to fill the room, within 3 days.*
>
> *The two elder sons could not decide what to do and spend all the time in thinking. The youngest son purchased a mud lamp, some oil and a little cotton. On the third day, he called his father to the room and lit the lamp; the entire room was flooded with light.*
>
> *The father was very much pleased with his wisdom and handed his business to the youngest son.*

Jealousy and comparison are like darkness that will disappear only if we bring the light of wisdom and understanding into it.

What is Proper Understanding:

1) Understand that each one of us is unique with a different agenda; there is no one like us in the entire universe. Then where is the scope to compare?

2) **Swami says:** In case we have to compare, compare ourself with ourself. i.e. Am I a better person than what I was 2…3…4… years back? This can be said to be a very healthy comparison, where we can keep on improving our own self by self- assessment.

Conclusion:

1) **Iccha Shakti (Power of desire and creativity)** is the energy that creates desires in us and this energy is potentially powerful enough to create **Kriya Shakti (Power of action)** to actually fulfill the desire created in us. This sutra is stated in the Upanishads.

2) As per the Upanishads, desires are energy forms. Without Iccha or desire we cannot get up or sit or stand or even move an inch. Hence desire is a basic energy of our life.

3) It is observed that every morning, **our desire to enjoy is the guiding force which makes our astral or mental body enters the physical body.** The desire could either be to enjoy something through our body or because of the fear of losing something, for example, we think that if we do not get up and go to work, we will lose our job, or if we do not get up, who will cook food for our family? The thought may not take this exact shape or form but it shows the **underlying insecurity, driven by fear or need or greed** that causes us to get up from our bed.

4) It is important to understand that we take human birth and are in bondage and keep going through the cycle of birth and death just to fulfill our desires. Our desires are the main cause for our bondage. So when we assume human form, we bring with us enough energy to fulfill those desires and to unfold those desires as well.

The **RISHIS (enlightened masters)** declare with conviction that, since we are God, if we have a desire, we have the power to fulfill it. Ex. If we have the desire to possess a house; the very desire can express enough energy to create the house in our life.

The **Brihadaranyaka Upanishad** says:- **as our desires are, so is our will; as our will is, so are our actions; as our actions are, so is our life.**

As all the Sahd Ripus are interlinked, the reader may find repetition in certain sections, such as material on **'gathered desires.'** We gather desires because of **Moha or attachment;** at the same time **Matshar or jealousy** is created because of gathered desires.

As we have just seen, desires are the cause of all the Shad ripus, let us now understand how to put a ceiling on these desires.

SAI RAM

'Ceiling on Desires'

"Man minus desire is God". Desires are what takes us away not only from God from our own peace, happiness and well-being".

– Sri Satya Sai Baba

7

Ceiling on Desires

The 'I' or Ego or Maya in us is created by God for **functioning** to happen and for the continuity of the creation. The Ego created the duality of '**me and mine'.** Because of this 'me and mine', 'you and yours', the functioning between individuals happens. This functioning creates **shad Ripoos** like Kama, Krodha, Lobha, Moha, Madh, Machar.

It is the 'I' who has desires and expectations. God has created this 'I' or Maya for relationships to function between 'I' and 'you' and because of these relationships there is continuity in the creation.

To survive on this planet earth, desires are required. The entire creation functions on desires and hope. The very base of all the desires is **Moha or attachment. Attachment** gives rise to **expectations** and **expectations** leads to **desires** and desires further leads to **Shad Ripoos. Thus we are trapped in a vicious circle, which again traps us in the cycle of birth and death, as birth is the result of unsatisfied desires.**

Some where we should stop this ongoing cycle of Birth and Death. Hence Swami teaches us to practice *Ceiling on Desires.*

How Desires Lead to More Desires?

DESIRES → EXPECTATION → fulfilled → more desires
↓
Unfulfilled → hope for next time so we pursue the desire.

So How to put a Ceiling on our Desires?

As Swami rightly says that there are five things which should be kept under control, in order to have ceiling on desires.

1) FOOD, 2) MONEY, 3) TIME, 4) ENERGY and 5) KNOWLEDGE

All the four are interlinked.

All our actions and function in life are based on the above five or rather life is a game we play with food, time, money, energy and knowledge.

a) Ex. To survive, **FOOD** is required. To buy or cook food, money, time, and energy is required. If we do not have the three we cannot get food.

b) If we do not have **TIME** we cannot enjoy food and money, for example, in office there is heavy work schedule and hence no time to enjoy money or food. Or has a lot of money but is sick with some chronic disease and cannot enjoy money or food hence no energy.
Ex. we have to catch a train and we are late. So we have to take a taxi instead of bus and spend more money and mental energy because of tension to catch the train.

c) If we have no **MONEY**, we do NOT get the proper type of food, hence no energy we get tired and work slow and hence lose time.

d) **ENERGY**: Time, money and food is another word for energy. If we have enough time we save money and energy. If we have enough money we have proper food and are not drained of energy and food gives us energy to survive. Hence all five are interlinked.

e) Without proper **KNOWLEDGE**, there are chances we cannot earn the money required and we waste more time and energy.

So when we have right controls and breaks on these five, automatically there is ceiling on desires, because without these five desires cannot be fulfilled. Control of senses also leads to ceiling on desires but to have control on senses, control of the above five things is required.

God has given everybody equal time, 24 hours a day and enough energy. How that time and energy is utilized properly to earn money and food depends on each individual. Further all the five i.e. food, time, money, energy and knowledge are useful and very important for our life to progress and evolve.

FOOD:

1) **Eat only when we need to eat** i.e. when we are hungry. Control our tongue when we feel like eating at wrong times.

2) **Always eat moderately.** The right intake or the best formula is – half of our stomach should be filled with food, 1/4th with water and 1/4th should be kept empty for proper digestion to function.

3) **Control of tongue is important.** Eating more food than required leads to diseases.

   Out of five senses the tongue is responsible, for us to curtail or control our desire for eating. Swami has told very beautiful things about the tongue which are as follows:

   a) The tongue does not loiter or roam here and there. It does not go to the other mouths; it remains inside, at home.

   b) When reading, talking or eating the tongue moves quickly from one side to another, forward and backward allowing the breath to come out as different sounds. It is so careful not to come in-between teeth like sharp merciless soldiers. Similarly we should watch all around to avoid danger and accident, not to fall in bad company or do not be led by bad habits etc.

   d) The tongue has no greed. If anything is good, it sends it down the throat to the stomach. If it bad or bitter it sends out and beyond the lips. It has no urge to have anything itself. It has no likes or dislikes. It's always clean. You must give up greediness. Do not get too fond of anyone or anything.

4) **Eating right type of food:** means eating **Satvik food** which gives us energy and is also good for physical and mental health. Avoid non-vegetarian food because it has bad effects on the mind, such as fear (animals that are slaughtered have fear and the same is carried in the food), animal qualities, lethargy and laziness etc.

Satvik food keeps our mind healthy and healthy mind has good and pure thought which leads to good actions. Hence Swami says 'Anam Brahman' – food is God so do not waste food. In India there are so many people who do not get food.

Hence practice Narayan seva. So do not take a lot of food in your plate (especially at marriage when it is free) and waste food. Hence right type of food, right quantity of food, eating at right times in a right mood will help us to keep ourselves fit and have ceiling on desires and also enjoy life in its right prospective.

TIME:

"Time Waste is Life Waste" "Time is God; don't waste Time"

Time is the most important needed factor of life, because everything in this creation is depended on time.

1) The main reason for man's birth and death is time. How? We do all our karma in time. To any event that has happened (past) or that is happening (present) or that will happen (future) we refer in time – past, present and future. The consequences good or bad that we face in day to day life are the results of our past karmas (i.e. in time). And the karma that we do in the present – good or bad will bear fruits in the future. Hence we are bound by karma which drives us in the cycle of birth and death.

2) Time is the main factor in our growth or evolution. If we waste time our life will be wasted. Do not degrade time by spending it in participating in unnecessary conversation or getting involved in others personal matters or no time should be wasted in evil thoughts and acts. Instead use time in an efficient way.

3) In actuality everything happens in the present. All actions or events happen in the present or Now and when we remember them we call it or recall it as the past. So there is no past. No-body knows what will happen in the next moment, so nobody knows the future. So everything is actually happening from moment to moment only. Therefore we should make the best use every moment of our life wisely for the moment which has passed will never come again.

4) When we hear a person saying that **he has no time** and yet he is interested in doing many things, what does it really mean? It means that **he does**

not have any more mental space to do any-thing more than what he is doing at this moment. The solution lies in creating mental space and not in blaming time ex. If a suitcase is to be packed with a lot of things, we have to iron and fold the clothes nicely so that the suitcase seems to take more capacity. The same applies to our mind and thoughts. The best way to utilize time is writing down our priorities. The secret of our success in any endeavor lies in the manner in which we determine our priorities to use time in an optimal manner. Anger is number one enemy of time. The greater the anger, the more the mis-management of time.

Swami says, in life, priorities should be: First God, second – the world and third – self. Then the time utilized will be the optimal

MONEY:

What is money?

Money can be said to be **Energy or Power** (purchasing power). Money is power which can make us its master or a slave.

Money helps us to satisfy our desires but does money give us happiness? Yes or NO?

It gives us happiness which is temporary and we desire and aspire for more. So what gives us happiness? **Contentment and fulfillment** which in other words is Lakshmi. In India money or wealth is considered as Lakshmi. In actuality Lakshmi means contentment or fulfillment.

Money can make you a slave to it.:

a) Some people call money bad. They say or believe that to have a lot of money is not good because it leads to wrong habits and vices.

b) When people have more money than needed they do not know what to do with it. As human nature is selfish (I and mine) and not ready to give easily; we start using it in a wrong way. We may spend money in unnecessary shopping, gambling, drinking, drugs and waste away our **TIME** and waste **MONEY** in wrong activities.

c) All this waste of **TIME and MONEY** is termed as **HAPPINESS.** But is there contentment or satisfaction? No. The more the money the more the desires. **All this leads to shad ripus due to lack of proper understanding.**

d) **More money leads to complexes:** Ego is boosted when a person becomes rich or has more money.

   He feels superior to others and has superiority complex. In very rare cases we find a rich person who is down to earth in temperament. Ex. Even when people give a donation they expect their name on the board of donors.

e) **More money leads to comparison:** which further leads to **jealousy.** People have a tendency to **show off.** This can be seen especially during give and take in at marriage functions.

f) **More money gives you position and power:** and with it more expectations. Ex. A well known dignitary in the spiritual field had visited Prashanti Nilayam. The management there were not aware of his status and he was made to sit in the public which made him very angry. Thus more money and power gives rise to ego which in turn gives rise to shad ripus if expectations are not met. (This happens only when there is lack of proper understanding).

g) Once the person gets the taste of power and position, he becomes **greedy** or **Lobhi** for money and wants more and more.

Thus all this is misuse of money which ultimately leads to the downfall of man.

Proper use of money: Be a master over money. Money as such is not bad, using your discrimination power and use money in the right way, this is very important.

1) **Use money when needed or required:** We cannot live without money. For all our requirements like food, clothing, shelter, travel, social obligations etc. i.e. to live a normal comfortable life we require money.

2) There is a very good principle among Muslims. Whatever they earn, 1/10th of their earning should be compulsorily donated for the welfare of the society. In the Khoja community they have a system of donating 1/10th

of their earnings to their community house or jamatkhana and also on occasions like birthdays, anniversaries or festivals they donate one person's food. Swami guides us as follows: 1/3rd of the earning should be donated, 1/3rd should be used as savings and 1/3rd should be used for our food, cloths and daily requirements.

3) In our shastra **Gupta Daan** is given very much importance. A lot of money is donated but no name is given.

4) When you help others by giving money, check that it is being used rightly. Example: If we have to give money to a beggar it is possible that instead of buying food, the beggar may go and drink alcohol. We feel we have helped the beggar, but instead we have spoiled his health and also put him in bad habits. Example: If we are helping a poor family to educate a child, see that the money is not used for social obligation. Instead we should personally pay fees or buy books etc. in this way money is put to right use.

   Ex. We give money to pay hospital charges and the same money is used to pay debts, so be careful where and how the money is used in case of individual help As in case of donations to trusts (which are most untrustworthy) be careful that you donate to the right trust as nowadays there are bogus trust with bogus receipt books to cheat the income tax department. So Swami always says that the ABC of life is Always Be Careful.

5) Giving or donating has its own importance. **There is a universal law.** 'As you sow so you reap'. If we sow one seed, we get a lot of grain from one seed. Similarly, when we give or donate we get back many-folds and the Creator's creation continues.

6) Swami says buy only what is required. Just do not go on buying because we have money. The same money can be used for a constructive purpose.

ENERGY:

What is Energy?

Energy is the essence of everything. Different names given to energy are power, shakti, urja, spark etc. Energy is God. How? Cosmic energy or Love energy.

Where is Energy?

Energy is everywhere, in all Panch Tattvas – Agni (inferno); Pritvi (Earthquake, gravitational force); Vayu (cyclone/storm); Jal (sunami/floods); and Akash (thunder and lightning).i.e. in the entire Cosmos.

Can you see Energy?

We CANNOT SEE ENERGY but we CAN FEEL ENERGY.

We can feel energy because it is the essence of everything. It is the abstract form so we can feel it. (experience it between both palms)

There are three different forms of energies, they are – Solid, (Physical), Liquid (subtle) and Gaseous forms. (subtlest).

Energy in Pancha Tattva

a) AGNI -   Electrical and Heat Energy. (Short circuit)

b) JAL -   Mechanical (in motion) and Sound Energy. Can be converted into Electrical energy.

c) PRITHVI - a) Earth – Magnetic Energy, Gravitational force.

   b) There is all type of energies involved in Matter. ENERGY IN MOTION IS MATTER. Every matter though seems solid and has a compact shape in which cells keep on moving. So in actual, nothing is solid.

   c) Earth or Prithvi has a power of Creation. (The result of two energies mixing is creation.)

d) VAYU -   Energy in Action – always moving hence mechanical energy and Sound Energy. Everyone knows the power of strong wind. It can create tornadoes, hence powerful energy. Strong wind uproots big trees, roofs of houses etc.

d) AKASH -   Sound Energy. Without space we would not have existed. To take any form space is required.

The Different Types of Energies

COSMIC ENERGY is the MOTHER of all Energies. All the rest of the energies are born of it.

1) Cosmic Energy
2) Magnetic Energy
3) Electric Energy
4) Atomic Energy-Cell Eng.
5) Electronic Energy – Atomic + Electric
6) Chemical Energy
7) Light and Heat Energy
8) Sound Energy
9) Kinetic Energy (motion in Relation to Force) In Greek Kinema or Kinemat means Motion.
10) Mechanical Energy

Uses of Energy

All the things or events that are happening are nothing but conversion of one Energy into other, resulting into creation of something new.

EVERYWHERE THERE IS COSMIC ENERGY OR LOVE ENERGY
(Light energy, God energy)
↓
SANKALPA -THOUGHT ENERGY - COSMIC MIND SOUND ENERGY OM
↓
ACTION-CREATION- MECHANICAL ENERGY (EKOHAM BAHUSHYAM) AND WE ARE BORN FROM THE COSMIC ENERGY.

Every-where there is Energy. The world is just a play of energy, the mixing of different energies to create something new.

Thought Energy can be positive energy or negative energy. Thought energy converted into word is sound energy.

Ex. – If people just abuse a tree it will die. (Word energy converted into action) Thought energy converted into action is MECHANICAL ENERGY.

Example of thought energy conversion of action – a) Zen masters practice the power of thought and can throw or drop a person with just a thought.

Love is a MAGNETIC ENERGY (power of attraction)

When positive and negative current meet ELECTRICAL ENERGY is created which further creates LIGHT, SOUND OR HEAT ENERGY (tube light, door bell, heating element).

Example: Left side of our body is negative and right side of the body is positive hence light or divine spark in us, because of which we have sight, sound and heat.

MAGNETIC ENERGY can produce currents or vibration to create ELECTRICAL ENERGY. Ex. Fan- Electrical – magnetic, mechanical and finally Air Energy.

Friction of 2 energies gives Electrical energy.

Ida (left nostril, cool) and Pingla (right nostril, heat) and Sahasrara chakra is the antenna. We take air energy while breathing and also get cosmic energy through the sahasrara chakra and this friction creates electricity in our body.

IMP: Like any other matter our body is made up of atoms and molecules. Each atom can produce 1/100 watt electricity (a torch has 1.5 watt). 40,000 watt electricity can be produced in 1square inch of human atoms. Ex. Sages had power to curse and burn things.

How Energy Affects Us?

Energy in Human Body – PHYSICAL, MENTAL and SPIRITUAL

PHYSICAL BODY: FOOD: All food is made of Pancha Tattva and also has all three forms, solid, liquid and gas. There are also positive and negative food items, example. Chillies are negative but Pepper or miri is a positive. Sugar is negative but honey is positive, i.e. they give us positive or negative energies.

The food passes from our mouth to different parts of the body because of Mechanical Energy. In the STOMACH there is JATHAR AGNI –ELECTRIC OR HEAT ENERGY

In our body different CHEMICALS are produced like saliva, hydrochloric acid, digestive juices and food mixes with these and CHEMICAL REACTION TAKES PLACE with the help of CHEMICAL ENERGY. And food is digested.

Various gases in the body (different Prana vayus) give Sound Energy: burping movement of gases in stomach which makes noises, passing of gas through the anus, etc.

Ultimately only the SATVA OR NUTRITON required by the body is distributed to the blood (Liquid form or Jal tattva) and to the body organs (solid form – Pritvi tatva) and waste matter is thrown out.

The waste matter too has energy which is again used as manure or soil and sometimes eaten by birds and animals (cocks, pigeons and pigs)

Conclusion:

Physical body has:

C E	Heat energy	-	Temperature of the body
O N	Chemical Energy	-	Different Chemicals in the body
S E	Mechanical Energy	-	Movements in the body.
M R	Atomic Energy	-	Blood and the organs have cells which takes the Energy
I G	Sound Energy	-	Various gases
C Y	Air Energy	-	Breathing –Purification of blood and removal of negative energy or waste products.

So we should understand that if we waste food or eat wrong food, waste water, agni (cooking Gas), etc. we waste energy. Over-straining and over-working also depletes our energy.

Mental Energy: Thought Energy

Mental Body through Chakras create an Aura round our body but a special Aura is around our head from ear to ear round which shows a Halo is the THOUGHT ENERGY – or MIND ENERGY which affects the whole body.

The Crown Chakra or the Sahasrara Chakra is open, and is always collecting Cosmic Energy from the Cosmos, which forms a perfect halo round our head. Our own thinking process affects this mind energy and this in turn affects the physical energy and health. POSITIVE THINKING STIMULATES it causing the energy to expand outward while NEGATIVITY draws the same energy downward eventually causing congestion throughout the body. Any Negative thought of anger, depression envy, jealousy etc. depletes this energy; a funnel is created in the Aura. This is creating unnatural pressure on the brain and if unchecked, causes congestion in the energy counterpart and alters the body biochemistry.

Mind energy stimulates the physical functions of the brain and the Mind energy expands and contracts as per our thinking. HENCE POSITIVITY BRINGS GOOD HEALTH. The collected thought energy passes through the crown charka or Sahasrara chakra and is distributed to the different chakras and in turn affects the various endocrine glands, which may create good health or bad health depending your thought process(positive or negative).

Another factor that affects the mind energy is the various types of shocks. A new born child comes to our dimension from other dimension. Its sudden entrance is a shock to it especially the light and sound effects on the child. This has an effect on the Energy body or the Aura of the child. Hence when a child is born, it should be lightly patted all over the body to bring back the Energy body into its original level.

Secondly the mother has to hold the child close to its body, so that it feels the same vibration when it was inside the womb, this relaxes the child and the energy bodies are balanced. It is observed that the result of such shocks is that child suffers from asthma, skin rashes or food allergies later.

Swami says: 'If you see bad things, your energy is wasted. Hearing bad things, speaking evil, thinking evil thoughts, and doing evil deeds are all waste of your energy'. Conserve your energy in all these five areas and make your life more meaningful.

The path of divinity is not seeing, listening, speaking, thinking or doing anything bad. If we are not following this path we are wasting our energy. On account of this waste of energy we are losing our memory power, intelligence, power of discrimination and power of justice. Hence do not waste your energies.

Knowledge:

Lack of use and misuse of **Knowledge** is one of the main causes of violence in the world today. Mere accumulation of knowledge or information, which is not put to use is like undigested food; not only it is waste but it also deprives someone else of benefit. Knowledge once gained has got to be used for the good of oneself and the society. The intention of acquiring knowledge is as important as the practical application to which it is put. By skillful use of the knife, the surgeon benefits the society while the same knife is used by a criminal for a violent act.

When we come to realize and practice by placing a **'ceiling on desires'** on our habits of self- indulgence, wastefulness, and greed, we move faster towards our goal of Self Realization.

Hence Ceiling on desires program is one that, man does not waste anything in the area of food, money, time, and energy and this is possible if we formulate and define our thoughts before they reach our mind. It urges us to practice self-restraint and self reform in our day to day living by turning our senses particularly the tongue, which binds us to our body and debases our nature.

Swami gives a very good formula that is to do everything in **moderation.**

When we are born there is no negativity in us (We are divine hence only positive), but as we grow we collect negativity, so our basic or original nature is positive. Any negativity causes disturbance in our physical and mental state.

So always BE HAPPY and FEEL HAPPY to keep yourself fit and healthy physically, mentally and spiritually.

Affirmation: I AM HAPPY, I LOOK HAPPY AND I FEEL HAPPY.

Here we have concluded the Chapter 'Yama', which is comprised of the six Shad Ripus and Ceiling on Desires. We now move on to our next Chapter **'Niyama'**.

SAI RAM

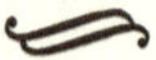

Chapter II

Niyama or Observance – Human Values

Satya	-	Truthfulness
Dharma	-	Righteousness
Shanti	-	Peace
Prema	-	Love
Ahimsa	-	Non-violence

NIYAMA:

The entire world is a combination of mind and matter. Man does not realize this and considering himself to be superior to it all. He is egoistic. He has forgotten his true nature. Inspite of undergoing much suffering, pain and sorrows, surprisingly man is still not ready and does not feel the need to know this. Nature is the combination of these two – mind and matter. When we realize the truth of what is mind and what is matter, we can understand the human nature clearly. The world is the expression of God's Will and creation is the manifestation of Gods will. This is called "Prakriti".

Everyone born in Prakriti should understand the nature of divinity. Man should express the divinity inits fullness.

"In this world every object has a value. The value of salt lies in its being salty. The Value of sugar is its sweetness. The value of fire is its capacity to burn. So every object has its own value. If that is so, has man no value?" Sri Sathya Sai Baba.

So let us examine the values of Man or Human Values

The 5 Human Values are **Satya, Dharma, Shanti, Prema and Ahinsa.**

All the 5 Human Values are very much interlinked. The reflection and the spark that has come out of love is called Truth. The same love when expressed in action is called Dharma. When love is contemplated upon, mind attains supreme peace. When we enquire from where this love has come and understand its source, then we realize the great principle of non-violence. **(Bases of Sadhana – Compiled From Divine Discourses of Bhagawan Sri Satya Sai Baba).**

The five Human values are like the five fingers of your hand and Love is the thumb in the hand. It sustains the other four.

As Swami rightly says that "Love is God, live in Love", we start with the first Human Value of LOVE.

Man is the form or spark of the divine. The Consciousness of man is God's will. All physical and mental energy's are forms of Satchitnanad. Therefore, all sankalpas of man are all sankalpa of the divine. This is called 'Prerana', the conscience.

The Conscience is called 'Sakshi Bhootham' a Witness. It is a witness to the divinity that is Love. (Bases of Sadhana – Compiled From Divine Discourses of Bhagawan Sri Satya Sai Baba).

SAI RAM

'LOVE' – First Human Value

"Love one another and help others to rise to the higher levels, simply by pouring out love. Love is infectious and the greatest healing energy".

– Sri Satya Sai Baba

1

First Human Value:
Love as Human Value

So we start with the 1ˢᵗ Human Value of Love. Being alive is itself a manifestation of love. Life begins with love, ex. We tend a plant, when the leaves are green. When the leaves dry up and the plant becomes a lifeless stick, we stop loving it. Love lasts as long as life last. Love is bound with life. Therefore love is life. The person who has no love to share is as good as dead.

The first that comes out of man is Love or Prema. He starts loving his mother, father, brothers, sisters, relatives, friends and prakriti or Nature. Thus life starts with love which is then expanded in our thoughts, words and actions.

The first feeling that came out of us is love and the same love is expressed in various ways, ex. Sugar. The sweetness can be felt in tea, coffee, biscuits, sweets etc.

What is Love?

1) Love is inherent **Divine Energy** verily present in everyone.
2) Love is a **radiation**, an illumination that comes from the inner depth of Consciousness of man.
3) Love is an **undercurrent** that flows through Sathya, Dharma, Shanti and Ahimsa. If thoughts are immersed in **Love, truth** will manifest in our heart. If our **actions** are suffused with love, then all our acts will exhibit **righteousness or Dharma.** If our feelings are soaked in love, we are able to enjoy peace, and if we are able to experience and understand the principle of love in all pervading nature then, **non- violence** will envelope us and

be present in all our endeavors. Thus love is the undercurrent of all values providing them divine quality.

4) **Love is the glue** that holds all atoms together, keeps planets in their orbit, and attracts one person to another. Love flows directly from the soul itself.

5) **Love is an indicator of Psychic development** of the individual. Where there is love, it means that a channel has been found for the soul to express itself. How?

Ex. If we see an old person suddenly falling on the road, what do we feel and why? We feel compassion (which is another form of love). Why should we feel this? The person is not related to us in any way, then why? There is some connection soul to soul and love and compassion is the channel.

a) How does Love become psychic development? Suppose the above scene is seen by a child of 9 month, 5 years, 10years, 18 years and 25 years. How will all of them react to the situation?

b) Degree of love and compassion from person to person indicates psychic development i.e. a person may just lift the fallen person and walk away. Other may make the person sit at side give water and the 3rd may hold the persons hand and help the person to reach his destination.

Types of Love

There are 2 types of love. 1) Selfish or worldly love and 2) Selfless or Atmic love.

1) **Selfish or worldly love:** Love that is related to the body has an element of selfishness. Any feeling of attachment to concepts, ideology, community or physical objects like property or a near relative is binding. **Sathya Sai Baba says: 'Properties are not Proper ties.'**

Worldly love tends to be conditional, restrictive, selective or transient. It always boost the Ego and the Ego always seeks its own benefit in all that it (ego) things, says and does.

2) **Selfless or Atmic love:** Love in its purest form is unselfish and unconditional ex. Mother's love for her child is a natural outflow from the very depth of the heart. It is energy that radiates from every cell in her body. Therefore mother's love for her off spring is the closest human approximation of

Divine Love. Divine love is expansive, pure, unselfish and liberating. The expression of selfless love is total giving without expectation.

Expansion is the essence of love. Ex. When a lamp is lit from another, the first one did not stop emitting light. You can light a million lamps from one, yet the first one will not suffer at all. Love too is like this, share it will a million, it will still be as bright as when it was alone.- Sri Sathya Sai (3rd March 1965).

Story:

A learned man once visited Emperor Akbar's court. In his speech, he praised Akbar sky-high, even saying that the Emperor was more powerful than God.

Akbar was amused. After the scholar had left, Akbar asked his ministers to tell him in what respect he was mightier than God. This put the ministers in a tight spot.

They could neither tell the truth, nor did they want to invite the displeasure of the mighty Emperor. When all were thus silent, Akbar turned to Birbal, "Birbal, at least you must have an answer". The jealous ministers were pleased, expecting Birbal to fail this time.

Birbal calmly replied, "O Emperor! It is true that at least in one respect you are more powerful than God. If you are displeased with anyone, you can drive him out of your kingdom. But if God is displeased with anyone, where could He drive them away?

God's Kingdom has no limits."

"NO ONE IS BEYOND THE BOUNDARY OF MY LOVE" –Sri Sathya Sai.

How to Develop This Selfless Love:

1) To develop such selfless love in our daily life, we should have co-ordination between Head, Heart and the Hands (3HV). The tongue may be considered to be the ambassador of the **Heart** communicating the messages, which originates from a thought (**Head**). The message should pass through three check points before it is communicated to others by word of mouth.

   The 1ˢᵗ check point is to answer the question, **IS IT THE TRUTH?** If the answer is approved then...

   The 2ⁿᵈ check point: IS IT NECESSARY? If the answer is affirmative then....

   The 3ʳᵈ check point: IS IT KIND and PLEASING? Upon a satisfactory reply, the tongue should utter the message. Thus harmony between thought (**Head**), word (**Heart**) and deeds (**Hands**) would be established. Baba always says 'You may not always be able to oblige, but you can always speak obligingly.

   Therefore the **spiritual practice for LOVE is Unity of thought, words and deeds**. Develop kindness, forbearance and forgiveness and discard selfish narrowness.

2) As Baba teaches, we should consider the faults of others, however big, to be insignificant. Consider our own faults, however insignificant to be big. Always remember that God is omnipresent. He sees and hears everything.

3) **Love grows by giving and sharing**

   o **GIVING:** Compassion, Sympathy, Helpfulness, Mercy etc.

   o **SHARING:** Egolessness, togetherness, affinity and identity.

   o **Giving:** It is good provided Ego does not pop up. In giving there should be an attitude of compassion, sympathy and helpfulness. In giving there is no one-way traffic.

   o **Sharing:** It is give and take. Hence, egolessness and a feeling of togetherness. When we share there is no feeling of high or low i.e. I am superior to the other and difference in status of society.

   o **Law of Nature:** What we give we get back but we get back 4 fold. good or bad. So, when we give, share with compassion, sympathy, mercy, togetherness, affinity, identity. There is a binding of Love and hence Love grows by giving and sharing.

4) **Understanding others promotes Love**

   When there is **attachment,** there is **desire** and if desire is not fulfilled it gives rise to anger, jealousy, greed etc. which pollutes the mind and hence no place for love. Ex. The burning charcoal of love does not glow when covered with the ashes of anger jealousy and greed. But when there is understanding which is a source of strength, leads to TOLERANCE and EMPATHY. Thus understanding leads to the growth of tolerance because Love is given from the source of strength rather than weakness (i.e. attachment, desire, anger, jealousy and greed). We may say attachment is a form of Love but it is selfish and love given with understanding is selfless. Thus we must transcend the physical and emotional obstacle and realize that **Love is powerful energy that can transform the hearts of others.**

5) **Patriotism**

   Expression of Love for one's country. Patriotism in real sense leads to self sacrifice ex. War heroes and freedom fighters. Panna dia – supreme sacrifice and Gandhiji's non- violent struggle for freedom is expression of Love deriving its **sustenance** from **Truth and righteousness.**

   Baba says – *Now- a- days, selfishness has taken place of self-sacrifice and Instead of patriotism i.e. love for country, politicians have selfish motto of position i.e. chair, name, fame and money.* How will patriotism help us in spirituality? Loving our country encompasses all our Country-men hence **expansion of consciousness** takes place. This makes us **selfless and egoless** which further leads us to our real self. Ex. Gandhiji was found counting matchsticks. When asked he said he was doing this to give mind some work so that it does not go haywire, and also to be in the present.

6) **Humanism**

   Through loving God, the next step is loving God in all men. **LOVE OF GOD EXPRESSES ITSELF IN SERVICE.**

When we do seva selflessly – we become egoless, there is expansion of Consciousness. When we do seva, the feeling of Love and gratitude and happiness you see in the eyes of other is in itself satisfying reward for the person who does seva.

Baba says – *'Love is God, God is love. Love more and more people; love them more and more intensely. Transform the love into service; transform the service into worship. That is the highest spiritual practice. (26th march 1965)*

Love springs from the heart when we are able to experience kinship with others ex. Million of cells in our body come to the aid of an injured part and help it regenerate the damaged tissue. The eyes shed tears of sympathy and the hand rushes for help. This show clear unity of human body and mind monitored by inner truth

Let us take the example of **a dot on a white paper.** What is it? We see the tiny dot and do not notice this whiteness all around. We tend to notice the negative and Ignore the expanse of light or Love that predominate. Actually, there is nothing evil in this world. All is pure and holy. Evil appears through faulty vision. If you have Prema towards all, everyone and everything appears suffused with Prema.

The mind sees separateness; Love sees unity. The only way the wavelet can know the ocean is to merge back into it.

Love is the fruit of life. The skin represents egoism, the 'I' feeling. The seed represents selfishness, the mine feeling, the possessive, the greedy, and the desireful principle. Discard this. What remains is the juice, the nectarine divine Love.

So **Swami says: Start the day with love; fill the day with love; end the day with love; this is the way to God.**

Truth is the current and Love is the bulb. Through Truth you can experience Love; through Love you visualize Truth.

So let us now understand the second Niyama – **Truth.**

SAI RAM

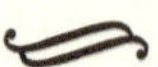

2

Second Human Value:
Sathya or Truth as Human value

Section I

The following explanation of Truth was given to me in my meditation on 12-10-2009, Monday.

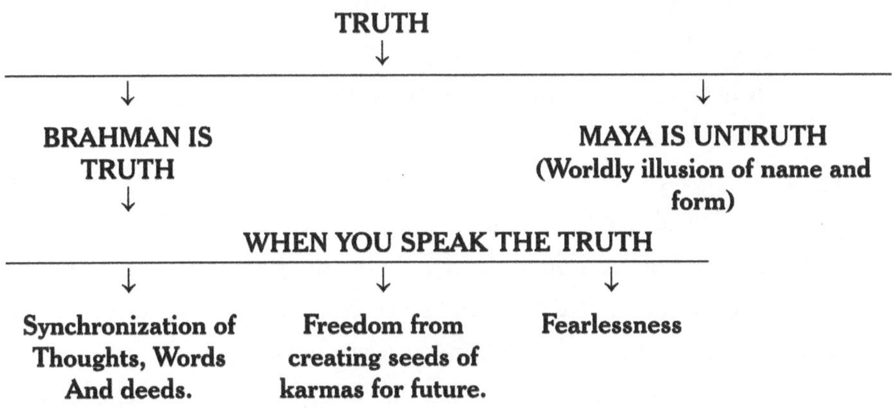

TRUTH:
What is Truth or Sathya?
Brahman is Truth – Conscious Level

Sat means – Being. Being is Consciousness and Consciousness is Brahman therefore **Truth is Brahman.** The entire Universe is nothing but Consciousness or Truth. It never changes, it is permanent or Nitya. Everything is just happening in Consciousness (i.e. all that we think, say and do is just happening in consciousness.

Another name for **TRUTH** is **SATYAM SHIVAM SUNDERAM i.e. Satyam means truth, Shivam means Consciousness and Sunderam means beautiful.**

Maya is Untruth – Ego Level

In Consciousness there exists illusion of name and form which we call the world. This world is not permanent and keeps on changing all the time, which is called **MAYA OR UNTRUTH.**

TO FUNCTION IN TRUTH / BRAHMAN / CONSCIOUS LEVEL WE MUST ALWAYS SPEAK THE TRUTH.

Benefits of Truth - or - When We Speak the Truth

1) When we speak the truth, we are functioning from our **Conscious level** or mode and not from Ego level or mode.

2) Truth remains the same in Past, Present and future while untruth may keep on changing as per persons and situations.

   Karmas are always created in Time. As truth is same in past, present and future it is **timeless** and hence **free from binding of Karmas**. So we do not create Karma seeds for future.

   In certain places or situations, you should use your discretion power, whether to speak the truth or not. In such cases one must keep quiet. So truth remains only at thought level and does not go to the emotional level and hence will not create guilt, and no seed for future Karmas is created.

3) When we speak the truth, we have no **fear** (fear of being caught). Fear is created by untruth and is done so because of Ego (which is also an illusion or false). So again we are functioning from the conscious level or mode.

4) **Satya Sai Baba means-** Satya means truth or being or Parmatma. Sai means Shakti or Prakruti and Baba means Shiva or Consciousness.

5) **TO FOLLOW TRUTH IS DHARMA AND DHARMA IS BEHAVIOR PATTERN**

Truthfulness or Satya:

1) Truthfulness means conducting our mind i.e. thoughts, speech and action according to truth.

2) Truthfulness is the result of our mind, speech and actions being unified and harmonious i.e. as Swami says 'Thoughts, words and deeds should be one!

3) Swami says 'Only TRUTH is non-changing i.e God. All the rest, the whole world is temporary and ever-changing. A proper understanding is required to understand this TRUTH.

4) There should be a realization that words which harm or hurt others are not truthful and if in speaking certain words someone is hurt then those words should not be spoken.

Truthfulness has 3 Levels:

a. **Thought or intellectual truthfulness.**

b. **Words or verbal truthfulness**

c. **Deeds/Actions or Physical truthfulness.**

1) **Thought or Intellectual truthfulness:** This can be practiced or lived if you have decided and accepted what truth is. When the intellect is dominated by inertia or passion the mind cannot discern between truth or untruth. The practice of truthfulness produces a steady mind and steady intellect which produces a steadiness in truthfulness upon which vocal and physical truthfulness depends.

 Example: When you have given your name for seva and because of laziness you give an excuse that you are not well.

 Example: You have decided to visit a close relative in a hospital with other members of the family and suddenly your friend comes with a good movie ticket, you select to go for the movie. This leaves a guilt feeling in you and whatever makes you feel guilty shows untruthfulness.

2) **Verbal Truthfulness (Vachika Satya):** It is only when we are established in intellectual truthfulness that we will be able to speak the truth. Speaking truth implies that we should speak that single truth that does the greatest good for the greatest number of people. Ex. False promises of politicians are good examples of verbal untruthfulness.

 Another aspect of verbal truthfulness is keeping one's word. There are times when because of karma, circumstance, devastation or other reasons, it is impossible to keep a promise you have made. So it is said that if a person at least has an intention to keep his word then he has adhered to truthfulness. So truth should be spoken only with wisdom, taking into consideration, time, place and circumstance etc.

Example: You had promised a friend to attend a function at her place but as you got ready to go, there was an emergency in the neighborhood and you had to rush your neighbor to the hospital which was a priority. In this case you had all the intentions to keep your promise but your duty or priority comes first and you call your friend and tell her the truth about the situation. Though you had all the intention to keep your promise, you could not do so.

Example: Sometimes it so happens that though you know the reality of a cancer patient, that he has only a few months to survive, you are helpless and cannot speak the truth. Instead you have to give him courage and tell him to chant Gods name as He is the ultimate healer. By saying so, you speak the truth and at the same time do not give false ideas of his getting well soon.

So here truth should be spoken with wisdom, taking into consideration, time, place and circumstance, etc.

3) **Action or Physical Truthfulness:** After the right thought and right word comes the right action. Truth must be unified in mind, speech and action. Physical truthfulness means good, truthful actions which uplift the mind and tends to lift the Pranic currents, extremely necessary for any one traveling the spiritual pathway.

Example: When you help some one, say, a blind man to cross the road, or some old lady who has slipped and fallen down on the road, how do you feel? The feel-good factor or the feelings of goodness that you experience will lift your Pranic currents in the mental body which is extremely helpful on your spiritual path.

The goal of Yama and Niyam is to reach a state of renunciation. Satya and Ahimsa are the keys by which this is done. However the importance of wisdom in observing truthfulness is equally important. How can Satya and Ahimsa be keys to renunciation? When we speak and follow truth we are always on the Conscious or Divine Level and when we function on the Divine level we automatically follow Ahimsa, which leads one to renunciation or detachment.

Swami Says:

> *Truth:*
>
> *Truth is unity of thought, word and deed. When action is saturated with Truth, it becomes Dharma. When all actions are right, peace reigns and one's mind is free from traces of violence.*

Most people have less understanding about the 'Absolute Truth'. They argue on the basis of scientific inferences. Therefore it is important to know the differences between scientific truths and absolute truth, that is to say difference between science and spirituality which we will understand in our next section.

NIYAMA: Second Human Value continued.....

SATHYA OR TRUTH AS HUMAN VALUE - SECTION II

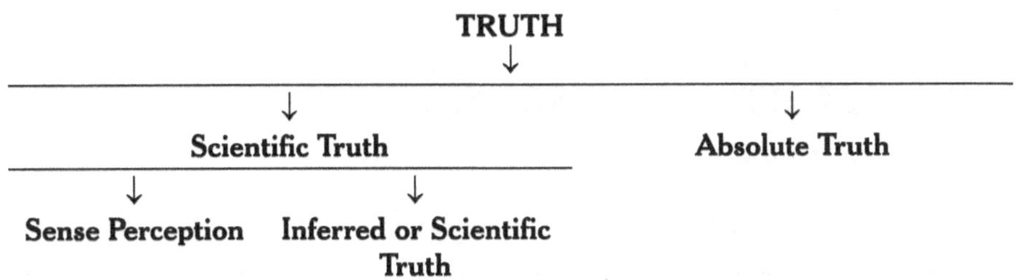

SCIENCE	SPIRITUALITY
a) Relative truth	a) Ultimate truth
b) Modified by time, space and gunas	b) Cannot be modified by time, space and gunas.
c) Temporary	c) Permanent
d) Knowledge of finite through sense Perception and Reasoning ex. Newton's Law of Gravitation.	d) Knowledge of infinite which has its own logic and Methodology.
e) Intellectual discipline	e) Intuitional discipline

f) Studies external (objective) world using senses and intellect which are subjective.

f) Studies inner life (Subjective domain), deriving inspiration from objective self.

g) Ex. Descartes, a French Philosopher said "I think therefore I am"

g) Upanishad sages have declared "I am therefore I think". For the essential is the Being.

What is Truth? Baba says "Truth has no limitations of time and space, for all countries, all climates, all times and everyone, truth is the same. Truth is changeless. So what is truth?

Truth is God.

Speaking truth in day to day life ex. Harishchandra, Mahatma Gandhi, WHY?

We hold on to truth with highest conviction that it proclaims our inner voice of conscious because of our faith in its infallibility.

So it is difficult to answer the question, What is truth? But we can understand truth if we know the levels of truth.

TRUTH BASED ON SENSE PERCPTION
What do we mean when we say "speak the truth?"

When we describe exactly what we see or hear, this is based on **Sense perception.** Sense perception truth varies according to time, location, situation and person.

Ex. Suppose, on the highway a serious accident has taken place. Mr. X sees the accident from the opposite side of the road. Mr. Y sees it from the car itself as he himself was in the car which met with an accident. Mr. Z was passing by in his car and observed the accident.

All three will describe the accident exactly as they have seen and heard. All are telling the **truth** but still it varies because of time, location (place), situation and person (each person has his own perception according to his understanding)

Therefore this truth is **Relative**. Fact and expression need not be the same and may differ from person to person. Hence this does not provide the whole truth, hence this truth is **temporary.**

A STORY:

The man had come to Mumbai, from the interiors of the state, with his two small sons for a holiday. Having heard so much about one of the renowned Amusement Parks, he took them one morning, wanting to give them a good time.

When he went to the ticket counter and asked for the cost of tickets, the man at the counter told him, that he would have to pay Rs. 150/-, while children above six years of age would have to pay the full cost those below six years were allowed at half the price.

The man counted his money, and found that he was short. He was about to turn back, when the man at the counter leaned out, and seeing the children, said, "If you say that the elder boy is not more than 6 years old, I will accept it, and charge you the half price for both".

The father thought for a moment, "No", he said, "I may tell you something that is not true and you may accept graciously, but in the eyes of my children, I would be a liar."

And he turned back.

INFERRED OR SCIENTIFIC TRUTH:

- It is at a higher level than sense perception. All scientific truths come under this category. Ex All men are mortals, sun rises in the east, crows are black, simple structure of Atom, 3 angles of a triangle add up to 180° etc.

- They cannot be **verified or demonstrated** under any circumstances. They cannot be observed by our senses, yet we accept them as truth.

- Through observation of events, collection of data is essential. A process of scientific reasoning is involved.

- Scientific truths are comfortably modified or extended in the light of new evidence, hence they are **relative truths.**

Absolute Truth or Divinity Within

Everything we see has the basis in the unseen, everything that we hear has a source which is unheard. Ex. Wall is seen but its foundation, which is its base is not seen in a garland the flowers are seen, the thread which is holding the flowers is not seen etc. Hence what then is the basis of Human body?

We say "my clothes", "my body", who is this **my? Who am I?**

The owner of the body, the master is the TRUTH declares Upanishads. The spark, flame is God, because He is the Source of All Truth and All Love. We may call it by any name like soul, Atma, Pure Consciousness or Divinity within.

Swami says "Man seeks truth. He seeks to know the Reality because his very nature is derived from God who is truth.

The Self:

1) Everything that happens i.e. raindrops we let pass by without concern, the artist draws, the poet composes, the musician sings, the peacock dances, the philosopher dream. **At the base of all this is the self (which is not seen).**

2) Self is self evident. No proof is required.

3) Not depended on logic and reasoning. Logic and reasoning flows from it. Other thing can prove and diagnosed, not the self.

4) The self which is the basis of everything is hidden within us. Swami teaches us that the process to uncover this hidden self is called is called **EDUCARE.** The word Education is derived from a Latin word EDUCARE

and EDUCARE means 'to lead-out or to draw out' that which is latent or hidden.

Swami Vivekananad's definition of education – 'Education is the manifestation of perfection already within the individual.

5) So we become aware of our true nature as perfection within us manifests with greater measure. To the sage, reality is not an illusion but a direct intuitive experience.

Truth is Eternal

1) At the highest level beyond time and space, self evident reality is common to all beings.

2) In this ever-changing world, the innermost source is the only permanent reality. What is God? or Self?

    The **Being** is the "Purusha" and Becoming is the "Prakruti" the ever changing world or Maya. The Purusha and Prakriti are 2 sides of the same coin and cannot be separated.

3) To understand and experience that the world is only **relatively real** is the path that takes us to the absolute. Each one of us take birth as per our Karmas and hence perceive the world differently. Each one's life is different and hence their experiences are different, hence the world they see is different. The world you see is real for you and the world I see is real for me.

"God is not high up in Heaven. He is in us, with us besides us behind us, before us. He is in every cell, in every atom as activity. He is all this and more besides. Every Human being is equipped with intelligence by means of which he can inquire, investigate and experience the central truth.- Sri Sathya Sai (18th August 1976).

The Hierarchy of Truth:

Every goal has a path with attainable milestones that lead up to it. Ex. While climbing a mountain, there are places of rest or another example is to get a post graduation degree one has to attain the mile stone of S.S.C. and Graduation. Similarly, truth has nine sub values (which are mentioned below).

These are based on Psychological principles. To each of the sub value one or more behavioral characteristic can be tagged. Every behavioral objective is an attainable mile stone on the path of Human excellence.

The sub values are as follows:
1) Truthfulness
2) Curiosity
3) Quest for knowledge
4) Spirit of Enquiry
5) Discrimination
6) Study of one's Self
7) Secularism
8) Respect for all Religions
9) Universal, Self-existent Truth

1) **TRUTHFULLNESS:** is in perfect accord with reality as perceived by the senses and implies correspondence between facts and its expression. i.e. when we speak the truth, the thought and speech are the same without any coloring of Emotions. **UNTRUTH** corrupts the mind, destroys its tranquility, pollutes the environment and harms the society.

2) **CURIOSITY, QUEST FOR KNOWLEDGE and SPIRIT OF EXQUIRY: - training the intellect:**
   The inner urge for self development leads one to ask questions, seek information and experiment. For this purpose we use our senses and also utilize our intellectual ability to think, remember and process the information to arrive at conclusion.

3) **DISCRIMINATION:** This ability helps us to distinguish between true and false, what is useful and what is not useful. This should be done with an open mind without prejudice, personal likes and dislikes. This is an important milestone along the path leading to truth.
   Man has to use the power of discrimination given to him to fight the evil forces within him, and to foster the divine elements in him by his own efforts, by listening to the voice of conscience – Sri Sathya Sai – March 1968

4) **STUDY OF ONESELF:** Now we are entering in the domain of subjectivity. The study of inner life requires the use of all the above steps, truthfulness,

training the intellect and discrimination. By making conscious use of the above we should do self enquiry as to 'Who am I" etc. collect information and investigate. At the same time we must strengthen our ethical and moral (conscious) behavior which is 'Swadharma'. This is very much required to awaken intuition.

How does this happen? When our behavior is one of 'Swadharma' and we behave as per our conscious voice within; there are no mental clashes and the mind is in peace, harmony which leads to intuition.

The real test is whether this will lead to internal transformation or merely picking of information to engage in unproductive dialogue.

Ex. If we want to see our reflection in the water, two essential conditions are applicable, firstly, the water must be clear and secondly the surface must be calm. Similarly to get into inner depths of one's own self it is essential to purify the mind (drive out all polluted thoughts and to quieten it (attain internal harmony and peace).

The real truth is the Consciousness. Words may be full of falsehood, but consciousness is always truth. When words follow the conscience then the words are also transformed into truth. (Sri Satya Sai – 13th January 1992)

5) **SECULARITY and RESPECT FOR ALL RELIGIONS:** Truth is only one. Truth that is the soul, atma etc. is one and the same in all.

All religions confirm the same truth and experience the same human qualities in all. Satya, Dharma, Shanti, Prema and Ahimsa are the basis of all religions. When we follow these it strengthens our belief in the brotherhood of man and fatherhood of God. This belief will not allow us to exhibit pride or prejudice in our behavior towards others.

There will be oneness which will expand our Consciousness and that leads us to the inner self or Truth.

Sri Sathya Sai Baba says: There is only one caste, the caste of humanity. There is only one language, the language of the heart. There is only one religion, the religion of love.

6) **UNIVERSAL SELF-EXISTENT TRUTH:** Our search for truth starts with, a conscious intellectual effort. Facts and expression should be same. The urge for self development (to understand the real-self i.e. Truth), there is curiosity, out of curiosity there is quest for knowledge and there is spirit of enquiry. The information gathered and experienced goes under the test

of Discrimination. All this leads to study of one self and while doing so you realize that all religions speak of the same Truth – brotherhood of man and fatherhood of God. Ultimately we understand that **TRUTH IS UNIVERSAL and SELF EXISTENT.** So the process (pursuit for truth) and the product (actual truth or the ultimate) merge.

Thus the enquiry begins with a conscious intellect effort on our part to search truth in the external world and fructifies with sublimation of intellect into intuition and outflow of love within us.

Swami says; **'Love as thought is Truth'.**

"The Universe is the body of God; every particle in it is filled with God, His glory, His might and His inscrutability. Believe that God is the inner Truth in everything and every being. He is truth, He is wisdom. He is Eternal. Sri Sathya Sai (20th May 1974).

Conclusion:

To conclude, all the nine sub values are interlinked and support each other. To understand the truth, we must make use of our full potential i.e. the faculties of head, heart and hand should be well organized. The intellect helps us to comprehend or understand through exploration, observation, analysis, interpretation and concept formation, the information gathered through self enquiry. Here memory is of great aid to compare and contrast the events and experiences with the knowledge within.

Following ethical and moral values promotes attitude development. This leads us to righteousness or Dharma.

So let's now understand Dharma or righteousness as the third human value.

SAI RAM

3

Third Human Value:
Dharma as Human Value

WHAT IS DHARMA?

Life is the game of the Divine. Just as any other game has rules and regulations to be followed for the perfect functioning of the game, similarly the game of life too has ideal set of moral restrictions and regulations which we define as **DHARMA.**

The Sanskrit word 'Dharma' has no equivalent word in English. The concept of Dharma goes beyond Religion, Righteous Action, a code of conduct, duty or obligation. Dharma means responsibility to self, others and God. It also means a number of fundamental principles that should guide mankind in its progress towards inner harmony and outer peace.

God created this world of His own initiative and ordained various codes for its upkeep and smooth running. There are rules of correct conduct for everything. These forms the Dharma – Sri Satya Sai (1966)

DHARMA AND NATURE

If we observe all around us, and understand the functioning of the entire universe and nature, we will agree that nature when left undisturbed is a perfect example of order, harmony and peace. It exhibits beauty and integrity in abundance.

We will observe that every single thing in the universe follows certain fixed laws of behavior or **Dharma.** The sun moves on its course with regularity, spreading its light and warmth to all without distinction. Water follows its dharma; its nature and obligation to move and wet; fire, the dharma to burn and consume. Fire cannot be called fire without its power of combustion and light. When it loses that, it becomes a useless bit of charcoal. The dharma of the magnet is to attract and draw unto itself. If it loses its power of magnetism, it will be a useless piece of iron. The Dharma of sugar is sweetness. If there is no sweetness, it cannot be sugar, but only sand. Every one of these is keeping up its Dharma, unchanged, including the solar system and the stars in the firmament.

Just imagine, what would happen if the sun failed to give us life-giving rays. It would be a crippled bee that did not share the nectar with the hive, or the fire refused to burn and give warmth. So too **we are the losers** each time we turn away from executing our duty gratefully and lovingly. Thus, Nature abides by the value of Dharma or Right Conduct in its physical expression, and motivates us to follow the path of Righteous Conduct, which is Dharma.

In short, that which is born in **Truth** is **Dharma,** that truth which is unchanging and permanent.

A STORY:

Once a wandering Sadhu reached the banks of a river, which he had to cross. While he was preparing to cross over to the other side, he noticed a scorpion

Struggling to get onto a floating leaf. In fact, it had almost drowned, but had managed to cling on to the leaf, trying to come on top.

Taking pity on the scorpion, the sadhu tried to lift it and place it on the leaf. Suddenly, the scorpion stung the hand of the sadhu, who withdrew his hand, and the scorpion fell off the leaf. The Sadhu saw that the scorpion was now drowning, but was trying to reach the leaf. The Sadhu, who was full of compassion, again tried to help the scorpion, and again it stung his hand.

> *Now, a passerby was a witness to the scene. He reprimanded the Sadhu,"Sir, you noticed how ungrateful the scorpion was in the first instance. Still, you assisted it the second time. Is this not a foolish act?"*
>
> *Still in pain from the two stings, the Sadhu replied calmly, "Your advice is well given, Sir, but the scorpion instinctively stung me. That is its nature. When the scorpion can stick to its **dharma**, how do you expect me to abandon **my dharma? (Swadharma)"***

All our functioning in our day to day life happens with the coordination of feelings, thoughts, words and deeds which leads us to right or wrong action so,

How to Follow Righteous Action, or Dharma

Righteous Conduct or DHARMA is the result of TRUTH.

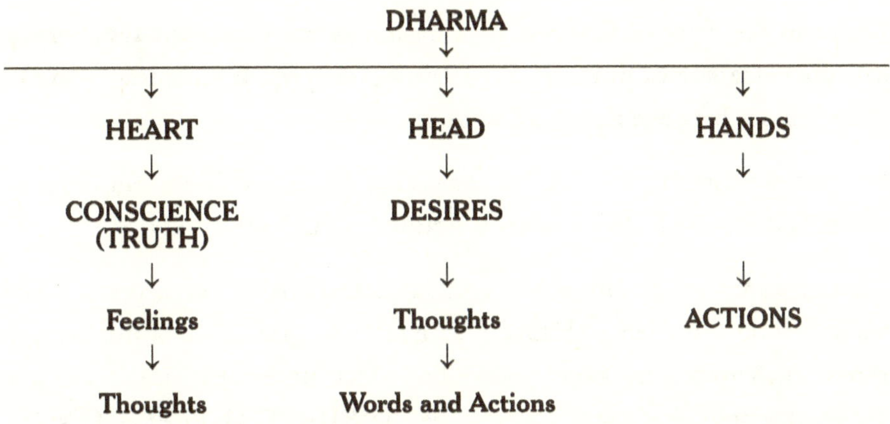

The entire Creation is nothing else but **Pure Consciousness** which is **Truth** and the **Conscience** which is in the **Heart** within us is the part of that Pure Consciousness which we call **divinity within us.** It is our guiding force and tells us what is right and what is wrong. It functions in the form of feelings, initially in an average person and when you are on the path of Spirituality and progress on the higher level; this conscience speaks to us as what we call the 'Voice of God' and guides us further in life.

The process of functioning in our day to day life in the external world starts with the five senses. The senses collect the data or information which gives rise to feelings. Most of the time, the data collected by the senses is a bundle of desires. Desires pull us towards the worldly objects, which is the source of worldly attachment. Hence the practice of **Ceiling on Desires** is important.

The **feelings** are then passed from the **Heart** in form of **thoughts** to the **Head.**

The heart represents our conscience and the head that is the thoughts represents desires. There is a tug- of-war going on within us between the voice of conscience and the attractions of the worldly desires.

When the voice of the conscience is subdued, the worldly desires take prominence and we fall prey to our self-created trap of the mind and follow the vicious cycle of insatiable desires and attachment. Hence there is disharmony and discontent all the time.

So my beloved Lord Sri Satya Sai (July 1974) says

Listen to the Voice of God within. As soon as one contemplates a wrong act, the voice warns, protests and advises giving up. It encourages you to discriminate between right and wrong.

So when we listen to the voice of conscience and follow it, we can never go wrong and there will always be right **Action** i.e. **HANDS.**

Thoughts are always expressed in words and then further into actions. When we follow the conscience (**HEART**), we utter or speak right words at right times. Such words are sweet and polite which never hurt others and the action that follows thereof will also be the **RIGHTEOUS ACTION OR DHARMA.**

Types of Dharma
There are two types of Dharma

a) Para Dharma or Worldly Dharma
b) 'Swa' Dharma or Atma Dharma

Bhagavad Geeta explains 'Swa' Dharma and Para Dharma. Brahmana Dharma, Kshatriya Dharma, Vaisya Dharma, Sudra Dharma are all worldly dharmas. 'Swa' has come from the Atma, Para Dharma relates to the body or Deha Dharma. In other words that which follows senses is Para Dharma and that which follows the conscience is Swa Dharma. We should always remember, whether the action is Swa dharma or Para dharma, that which is born in Swa dharma or Conscience, is very important for our life.

Understanding Dharma in the Right Sense

Sathya or Truth is the law of the universe and dharma is the path. When we become aware of Truth or at least some aspects of Truth, we start functioning from the level of consciousness or awareness. Speaking truth is utterance of what we think and dharma is acting according to our words. Here the unity of thought, word and deed is essential.

The first thing to be practiced is what we teach or advise others, we should practice ourselves. That is true dharma or humanness. All human values are contained in every cell of the body or else we cannot be human. We must understand what humanness is and practice it.

Unfortunately, the world is full of people with the attitude of 'I' i.e. Ego or Ahamkar,

'Me' and 'Mine' i.e. the Mamakara and Abhiman or Pride. This has risen from the physical and mental faculties and wealth. All the three are worldly in nature and have arisen because of relationship. So even in the epic of Mahabharat, Krishna advises Arjuna to give up Abhimana. So we should have Atma Abhiman and not deha Abhimana. All the three are just illusions and hide the real humanness, which is your real dharma.

How to Practice Dharma

Each profession has a Dharma, a set of moral restrictions and regulations guiding its exercise; if these are honored, then the joy of the participant will go on adding itself. The Dharma for each has to be different for it is

decided by changing factors like age, profession, authority, scholarship and also by considering whether a person is male or female, teacher or pupil, master or servant, child or youth, father or son, dependent or free. Sri Satya Sai (18th May 1968).

Performing our duty well results in true happiness in life and hard work done to fulfill our obligations yields the greatest satisfaction.

Our duties depend upon our circumstances. Some duties are to ourselves and some are to others.

In young age it is appropriate to work and earn a living and gain wealth and fame and also a well established place in society, as long as we have honest intentions to achieve them. In youth we have family and social responsibilities. However, when we reach an advanced age, we have the duty of detaching from the worldly affairs and fulfilling our spiritual goals.

No work is small or unimportant, do well. All the work that is given to us by the Lord is to enable us to reach spiritual fulfillment. There is no differentiation between God's work and our work. All work is God's work and it is not possible to separate the temporal from the spiritual.

Sometimes circumstances are such that it is beyond our control and we are called upon to perform certain duties. Our freedom to select or choose our course of action could be limited. One individual may have a greater freedom to choose the path of action than the other whose opportunities are restricted. Hence immediate results of our actions are less important than the motive behind them. We must do our duties to the best of our ability and leave the results to God.

While performing our duties or Dharma, attachment to the self has to given up and all the acts have to be performed in a spirit of worship and dedicated to God. While performing our duties we have to see God in every man. We have to give up the idea of doer-ship, that we are the doers. In actuality, neither do we do any-thing nor does anything belong to us. God himself is the writer, producer, director and actor of the Divine play of creation. Hence we have to perform all our duties with the attitude of surrender and drop the idea of doer-ship, which is just an illusion.

A person who follows Dharma cultivates good conduct and character and proves a good example to society. Further he should also imbibe the four noble qualities of Self Confidence, Self Satisfaction and Self Sacrifice which will ultimately lead him to Self Realization. These four form the sub-values of Dharma.

Man allows the mind – a mere bundle of thoughts and desires – to guide his ACTIONS, instead of the faculty the intellect, which can discriminate, probe and analyze. But the mind follows blindly every whim and fancy. The intellect helps one to identify ones duties and responsibilities.

– Sri Sathya Sai (13th April 1981)

The 4 Sub-values of Dharma

The four sub-values of Dharma, mentioned above are to be inculcated from a very tender age. To repeat them, they are Self confidence, Self Satisfaction, Self Sacrifice and ultimately Self Realization.

When we internalize these values they are reflected in the conduct and are observed by others. At a very early age, children have to be taught certain mannerisms which form into a habit with regular practice. They are:

1) Cleanliness and hygienic living which includes regular bath, brushing teeth, cutting nails, grooming of hair, good eating habits.
2) They should also be taught time management; how regularity and punctuality lead to better utilization of time; the importance of simple living and high thinking.
3) Next they should be taught to be self dependent; that is to do things on their own as appropriate to their age for example, Keeping their books and other things properly in place, doing homework on their own and acting responsibly in carrying out small tasks assigned to them all lead to self- reliance. All these habits give the child **Self-Confidence.**

As the child grows, this Self Confidence helps the child to interact with the social environment in a meaningful way. Obeying and respecting elders, respecting others' ideas and views; when working as a team, the child inculcates team spirit and dignity of labour etc. He also finds doing duty and service to others, a fulfilling and rewarding experience. Thus functioning in society provides him **Self- satisfaction.**

Along with the social interaction, the guidance and the encouragement given by the Parents and teachers, strengthens the will of the child. This generates worthy attitudes such as honesty, resourcefulness, initiative, courage, leadership, justice and faithfulness, while functioning in his day to day life. This brings about internal transformation, which prepares the person for **Self-Sacrifice.**

Ultimately when the child grows to become an adult, all the above qualities inculcated by him in early childhood leads him in two directions simultaneously.

1) Interacting with the social environment and
2) An exploration of the inner life.

They understand life better, and become good human beings. The more they dwell deeply within themselves, the more effectively they will be able to exhibit Dharma in real life. Following the path of Dharma and with all the above qualities, will lead us to the end goal of **Self-Realization.**

When we follow the path of Dharma or righteousness, there is less agitation in our mind which finally leads us to experience peace. So let us understand, the next Niyama – Peace or Shanti.

SAI RAM

4

Fourth Human Value:
Peace – Shanti

WHAT IS PEACE?

Peace is the most priceless possession of man. It is our real nature. It is futile to search for peace outside. Peace is found within. Peace is a state of mind or Consciousness which is achieved when we merge with the Source. We are like musk deer running frantically in search of fragrance that fascinates it and when it gets too exhausted to continue it discovers that the source of fragrance has been within itself all along.

Agitation in the mind is the cause of all misery of mankind. When the mind gets agitated we lose peace.

Today we live in the world full of disputes, fights and wars. Absence of war is hailed as peace. Such peace is superficial and termed as cold war. Inaction is not really a sign of peace. It is peaceful in the cemetery. Can we call that peace? We feel disturbed even in a static situation.

Control the Mind and We Remain Unruffled, This is the Secret of Peace.

A STORY:

Once a rich man came to Swami. He looked very disturbed and unhappy, despite his fame and wealth. With a great feeling of distress, he pleaded with Swami saying, "Baba! I want peace."

*Swami looked at him for a moment and said, "Ponder over the three words, **I want peace.** The answer to your prayer is hidden in the three words. Remove the "**I**" feeling, the root cause of this "**I**" feeling is the ego. The "I" will persist as long as you are embodied, but try to minimize its hold on thought, words and deed. **Want.** Want to possess, to acquire, and possessing has no limits. The more you possess, the more you desire. Reduce and eliminate your wants. Now, when the "**I**" and the "**Want**" are taken off, what remains is '**Peace**'."*

To control the mind, we should know more about the functioning of the mind. The mind can be divided broadly into 4 stages or levels.

Stages or Levels of the Mind

1) **Conscious mind, 2) Sub Conscious mind, 3) Unconscious mind and 4) Super Conscious mind.**

Conscious Mind

In our day-to-day life we gather information of the world around us through the five senses. 83% through eyes and 11% through the ears. The information enters the body and is carried by the nerves to the brain where it is processed. The conscious mind then becomes aware of the information. As a result of the stimulus received from the senses, thoughts occur in the conscious mind. Each thought is a quantum of energy. The information in the form of thoughts is then send to the sub-conscious mind to be stored in the memory. Ex. Walking: conscious Mind - decision to walk. sub conscious Mind, directs the muscles to walk.

Ex. Eating of food – conscious mind and digesting of food – sub conscious mind. Ex. Sometimes we forget simple names and when we start thinking consciously it suddenly springs from the memory (sub. conscious mind)

Now we have a **CHOICE** to make about what is good for us. All things in our mind (Box) may not be useless. So learn to select the right thoughts.

Subconscious Mind:

The sub conscious mind is called the lower mind. It is a humble servant and **executes** all the decisions taken by the conscious mind without questioning. Sub conscious mind does not do anything of its own. It does what it is told to do. In sleep, the conscious mind does not function but the sub conscious mind works and hence all body processes go on.

Dreams and Memory is a part of sub conscious mind. Sub conscious mind influences our conscious mind because of our habits and experiences and traditions stored in memory (conditioning and traditions of the past years).

As the information is received and stored in the memory, the sub conscious mind compares and contrasts this information with the impressions of the past. If it finds the information negative then it will send a negative emotional reaction back to the conscious mind, which will respond with anger, fear etc. If it finds the information positive then it will send positive emotional response to the conscious mind which reacts with pleasure, joy, excitement etc. In both cases the response of the sub conscious mind is again stored as content of past impressions. Hence the Sub Conscious mind is the sum total of all our past experiences and hence we tend to regress into the behavior pattern of the past.

It is generally believed that all our effort should be directed to satisfy our many desires in order to attain peace of mind. Desires are a chain of thoughts and arise when the mind craves for experience which has to be gained through our senses. Our desires are never ending and our mind is never satisfied. If one desire is satisfied the other bounces back with greater intensity. Outward means to satisfy the mind only increases the agitation of the mind.

Giving free play to the senses just because they belong to you is foolishness. Although it may be your horse, you do not let go the reins, while riding; you will meet with disaster. Similarly you may say 'it is my car', but if you do not apply brakes where necessary, even though it is your car, it will lead you to danger. Sense control is thus imperative for all human beings not just for saints and seers – Sri Sathya Sai (1979).

As stated above, the horses are the senses and the reins are the mind; if we do not hold the reins in control the horses will gallop freely in all directions and led to our destruction. Hence the mind has to be trained to obey the command of the intellect.

How to Attain Peace

All the consequences of our past experience is stored in us as emotions; hence they cannot be erased. When the intellect takes charge with full awareness, it becomes possible to maintain our balance, our peace of mind. We should consciously minimize negative thoughts and experiences and train the mind in positive thinking. When we repeatedly do something, it becomes conditioned in the sub-conscious mind; then this conditioning takes over and habit is formed. We must be constantly aware of this integrated relationship while reinforcing positive tendencies.

With the help of intellect we should develop proper understanding to control the emotional outburst pouring from the sub conscious mind. As long as the mind is involved in worldly desires we experience pleasure and pain, happiness and suffering, alternately all the time. Since it is difficult to eliminate desires totally, we should convert our worldly desires into spiritual desires, for truth, for God. Then the conscious mind will take its advice from the higher mind or the **Super Conscious Mind.** For this to happen we have to develop love for all. Our thoughts, words and deeds must be filled with Pure Love. This should reflect in our day-to-day behavior. Only then we will be free from the dominance of the mind and the senses.

The Super-conscious Mind

The super conscious mind is the ultimate **PURE CONSCIOUSNESS.** It is the **Conscience,** the divinity within us. It is the Truth, the **Atma.** This part of the mind contains all knowledge and wisdom. Since Love springs out from the truth, the super-Conscious is also called the Spiritual Heart. It is in this region of the Self that our search for peace ends. Once we settle down in the Super Conscious mind, there will be peace. The mind will become calm and pure.

Experiencing Peace

Peace is an elevating experience which comes when one attains merger with the very source of one's Being. This state of mind is not the result of frustration. It bestows on us the capacity to bear success and failure, joy and misery with equanimity, which the scriptures call **Stitaprajnata** or **equal mindedness.** This state is such that we do not get upset with disappointments nor do we feel elation with success. There is a deep contentment with whatever happens around us. **Peace is power-packed stillness based upon contentment, self-confidence and self-awareness.**

I WANT PEACE, consider this statement. Sri Sathya Sai says, if you seek PEACE, cross out the 'I' and the 'WANT'. The 'I' represents the Ego i.e. identifying with the body and mind. When we identify ourselves with the body and mind, we break our contact with the self and lose peace. The function of the Ego is to establish worldly relationships and desires are the causes for WANTS. When 'I' is cut and desires or wants are reduced, Peace is definitely attained as our natural birthright.

Global peace is directly dependent upon peace in the individuals. As Sri Sathya Sai says:

If there is righteousness in our Heart
There will be beauty in character;
If there is beauty in character
There will be harmony in the home;
Where there is harmony in the home
There will be order in the nation;
And when there is order in the nation
There will be peace in the world.

When there is peace in the mind; non violence follows automatically. Non violence is the result of the peaceful mind. We will be able to understand non violence better when we explore our last Niyama of non violence.

SAI RAM

5

Fifth Human Value:
Non-violence or Ahimsa

Today we are living in the world of violence. Everywhere in the world you hear of fights, wars and disputes. The conflict is not only between man and man but also man and nature: we have not spared even the mother earth. Chemical pollution of rivers and sound pollution in cities have reached alarming proportion. Destruction of forests and exploitation of other natural resources has brought degradation to the earth's biosphere. There is no objection to man's enjoying natural resources. It is because of greed and uncontrolled desires and reckless exploitation of natural resources, that nature is exhibiting disorders like earthquakes, volcanic eruptions, Tsunami, drought and floods. Therefore the natural universal law 'You sow as you reap' applies here very well.

Mankind today appears like a foolish man who is wielding an axe at the branch of the tree on which he is sitting.

MEANING OF AHIMSA

Another Golden Rule we should strictly follow is 'Do not do to others what you do not like to have done unto you.' The true meaning of Ahimsa is not to cause hurt or harm to any living thing either through thoughts, words or deeds. Every action of ours must be examined before execution to see that we do not cause pain to others.

Non-violence is recognizing the omnipresence of God in every living thing. He is equally immanent in every living being in equal measures. So man should neither harm others nor be afraid that others would harm him. This is the philosophical basis of the Indian ideal of Ahimsa.

When we see oneness of all creation, it helps the flowering of non-violence in our thoughts words and deeds. When we thus follow non violence there will be the right understanding that all humans, animals, plants, lakes, mountains and glaciers are inseparable parts of the one indivisible Supreme Absolute. When there is feeling of oneness there is love. Hence **Love + Understanding = Non- Violence.**

There is Unity in all Creation. We can see this by referring to our own Physical body.

When your teeth bite your tongue, you do not punish your teeth. The right hand will not bring any pain or harm to the left hand unless it is our utmost necessity in the interest of the whole body. If a thorn pricks our left hand, the right hand will immediately come forward to remove it. It is the eyes that shed tears when a foot is injured although a great distance separates them and they have very different operations to perform. Just as there is unity in the whole body similarly there is unity in the entire creation. When we understand this unity, we will understand the value of non violence which takes us on a voyage from 'I' to 'WE', realizing that we are a part of one big family.

God is Omnipresent. He is immanent in every being in equal measure. So, man must visualize Him equally in himself and in others. That is to say, he sees God in all. So how can he injure others or fear that he will come to harm through others? This is the basis of the ideal of *Ahimsa* (Non violence). – Sri Satya Sai (14 November 1995)

The Practice of Non Violence

The observance or practice of Ahimsa in thought, word and deed is very important.

Non Violence of Thought or Intellectual Level

Complete non violence involves the renunciation of violence in body, in speech and especially in thought because the main source of non violence is within the intellect. Never think of hurting others, or criticizing or condemning others. Do not forget that whatever you face in life are reaction, reflection and resound of your own inner thinking. The thoughts or energies in the mind may be harmonious or inharmonious, which is ascertained by the intellect, and later these are manifested as actions. Hence controlling the mind or thought is the first step in the practice of non violence. This is also called Baudhika Ahimsa.

Non Violence of Word or Speech Level

When the mind or thoughts are mastered, you have mastered intellectual non violence. When this happens, non violence of speech or word becomes perfected. In practice, you must be very careful about your speech. Man's greatest weapon of offence is his tongue. The wounds that the tongue inflicts can be more severe than the damage caused by an atom bomb. Loud talk, insulting statements, talk full of anger and hate, wild talk – all affect the heart of man.

Verbal non violence arises by acquiring the verbal habits of Speaking softly, gently and wisely. The less you talk, the sweeter you talk, the better it is for you and the world. Perform all your acts with minimum noise and transact all dealings with minimum speech, for loud noise adds to the noise pollution and is sacrilege to the akasa.

Hence Mahabharata rightly says that the wound caused by arrow or axe heals swiftly but a wound caused by violent speech heals very slowly.

Non Violence of Physical Action

Physical non violence means not cutting, wounding, bruising or killing any other body or one's own body. Very often we do violence to our own body through improper diet and our wrong ways of living. Once we are established in intellectual and verbal non violence, physical non violence is also established.

It is important to understand intellectually and spiritually that the same spirit pervades in all life. The spirit in the elephant is not large nor the spirit in ant, is small. Hence dignity of your being is dignity of every soul.

In the practice of non violence, the grosser manifestations should be controlled first. To start with physical violence, killing, striking or hitting etc. should be controlled first. After this has been mastered, tongue control should be practiced, by not speaking cutting or hurting words. Lastly, control of thoughts, moods and attitudes must be mastered.

The above processes are not one-two-three processes. They are interrelated and interact with each other.

Non violence can be practiced by steadily limiting the extent to which we satisfy our many desires. We should regulate our use of food, money, time, energy and knowledge. The root cause of violence is the proliferation of desires. When we practice Ceiling on desires on our habit of self-indulgence, wastefulness and greed, we are able to reduce acts of violence towards all living forms and the whole environment.

A STORY:

During the early days of research on the sensitivity of plants, Dr. Jagdish Chandra Bose, one of India's foremost scientists in the twentieth century, uses to walk along a garden path, from his house to the laboratory and back.

Along the path, was a plant of 'touch me not,' which reacts by closing its leaves, when anyone touches the plant. This is its nature. Dr. Bose pondered over this phenomenon.

Once, he decided to try an experiment. He stood near the plant, and said loudly, "O beautiful plant, please have no fear from me. I love you. I want you to prosper. In fact, I will protect you, if necessary. Let us be friends. Have no fear on my account." Thus everyday he used to repeat this with a feeling of love, each time he passed this plant. A few months passed.

> *One day, the scientist observed that the plant did not withdraw and did not close its leaves upon his touch. This was his greatest moment of joy!*
>
> *So when you have no intention to harm others and have only pure love in your heart, then even the nature responds.*

The Benefits of Practicing Non Violence

1) When you practice non violence sincerely, it magnetically and mystically draws into your life non violent people and events. Your social exchanges become filled with happiness and pleasure and there is an effortless intellectual exchange and exploration of human consciousness. The more you realize that the same Atma or divinity is in everything, the more easily you become established in non violence You are not disturbed even when someone hurts or insults you and this brings about an unscattered mind and peace reins.

2) It brings about accumulation of good karmas in this life time as well as succeeding life times.

3) The mind is calm, there is no agitation and irritation of the mind. So concentration is possible because of which meditation happens and illumination is possible, which helps you to attain the goal of life.

According to Yoga Sutra, when a person becomes completely established in non violence, violence cannot touch him. Non violence is a great and noble state which few are capable of attaining for example, Mahatma Gandhi.

One important thing to be noted is, all the rules laid down by Yama and Niyama must be according to CLASS, TIME, PLACE AND CIRCUMSTANCE. A person must understand well these four conditions in order to live a spiritual life in the physical world. In the practice of non violence killing is not permitted yet it is quiet proper under certain circumstance to defend a child against a wild animal.

To a yogi living in an ashram or monastery or cave these rules are to be strictly followed but for a householder these rules are modified. A householder is permitted to burn logs, oil or coal for cooking, though in doing so one may destroy the insects living in these natural products.

The best way to practice non violence is to follow the path of Dharma according to our station in life and our spiritual understanding. The intention and our attitude to refrain from violence and carefulness in living is what is important. We must always weigh and balance the pros and cons before participation in any given action, so that we do not harm or hurt anyone.

It is of paramount importance to understand that non violence stems out of strength of human character, not an act of cowardice. It is much easier and perhaps 'natural', to hit back when one is stuck, but it takes tremendous self-control and courage to remain calm and unaffected. It is an even greater value to be filled with love all the time. To love others as oneself and to understand all creation as One is true non-violence.

All the five Human values of Satya, Dharma, Shanti, Prem and Ahimsa are the qualities of our inner divinity. They always exist in us. By practicing them we bring and express these qualities in the outer world and prove that we are Divine Beings in human forms.

By the regular practice of Yama and Niyama, there is a complete transformation in our thinking pattern and this in turn brings a complete change in our attitude. This positive change helps us to move to the higher level of consciousness, on our journey towards the ultimate.

To bring this change of attitude, we require a healthy body and mind. Let us discuss in the next Chapter of Asana, how practice of Asana helps us to keep our body and mind fit and fine.

SAI RAM

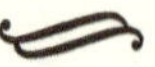

Chapter III

Asana –
(The Classical Postures)

WHAT IS ASANA?

Asana means a state of being in which we can remain calm, quiet, steady and comfortable, physically and mentally. 'Yoga' means experience oneness or unity with our inner being. This can be achieved after dissolving the duality of mind and matter into the supreme reality. In 'Yoga Sutras' an ancient text by Patanjali, Yoga asana means Sthiram sukham asanam which means the position which is steady and comfortable. Basically the practice of Yoga asanas is to develop the ability to sit in one position without discomfort for a longer time, as this is necessary during meditation.

Swami in his book 'Dhyana Vahini' gives a very good example of why asana is important. He quotes **'With the loins girded, the sleeves of the shirt rolled and the palms rounded into fists, it is not possible to exhibit love or devotion. With bended knees, the eyes half-closed, and the hands raised up over the head with the palms joined, is it possible to show one's anger or hatred or cruelty? That is why the ancient sages (rishis) use to tell the spiritual aspirant that it is necessary during prayer and meditation to adopt an appropriate bodily pose. They saw that it is possible to control the waywardness of the mind by this means.**

Until the goal of Meditation is achieved, the well established discipline of sitting postures (asanas) has to be followed. (Dhyana Vahini – Chapter II - Page 15 and 16).

History and Mythology

The Science of Yoga along with Asanas is said to be found in the oldest literature of mankind, the **Vedas** composed by realized rishis and sages of that time. Many statues have been found depicting Lord Shiva and Parvati (his consort) performing different yogasanas in the archaeological excavation made at Harappa and Mohanjadaro which is now Pakistan. The ruins were once the dwelling place of people, who lived in the pre-Vedic age, even before the Arayan civilization flourished in the Indus valley subcontinent.

Lord Shiva is the founder of Yoga, including asanas, as per scriptures and tradition. He created all the asanas and taught them to his first disciple, Parvati. It is said that originally there were 8,400,000 asanas which represent the 8,400,000 incarnations every individual must pass through before attaining liberation from the cycle of birth and death. Throughout centuries, rishis have modified and reduced the number of the asanas to a few hundred. Out of these only 84 are discussed in detail, and only 30 or so are commonly thought of as being useful to modern man.

Yoga is the offshoot of Tantra. Tantra is a combination of two words, tanoti and trayati which means respectively 'expansion' and 'liberation'. Therefore tantra is the science of expanding the consciousness and freeing it from its limitations. Parvati is regarded as the mother of the whole universe and is the embodiment of supreme knowledge. By her grace a person becomes liberated and is united with the supreme consciousness (Shiva). Out of love and compassion for all her children she imparted her secret knowledge in the form of tantra shastra. So we cannot separate Yoga from Tanta; both come from Shiva and Shakti.

The great Yogi Goraknath was the first historical exponent of yoga asanas. He taught all the asanas to his disciples. In those days the yogis lived in the mountains and forests, where they led a life of seclusion and austerity getting all their support from nature. Animals were the great teachers of these yogis for they lived a natural life free from disease and worldly problems. Animals do not visit doctors, their only help is nature. Many yogic techniques were developed by studying birds and animals in the forest.

For example; Kukkutasana (cock), Simhasana (lion), Mandukasana (frog),Gomukhasana (cow), Matsyendrasana and Matsyasana (fish), Makarasan (crocodile), Mayurasana (peacock), Vrushasana (bull), Garudasana (eagle), Vrukshasnan (tree), etc.

Comparison Between Yogasana and Other Exercises

Asanas are specific body positions to maintain physical and mental steadiness. They cannot be compared with gymnastics or body building exercises, nor can they be compared with modern day aerobic exercises. In gymnastics more importance is giving to developing the muscles and shaping the body by stretching and tensing the muscles and nerves. This seems to look good when young but they bring a lot of problem in old age when you stop it. Similarly the aerobic exercises consist in speedy and forceful movements of the body. Both the above mentioned exercises are responsible for making the mind extrovert and develop a challenging spirit. There is no rhythmic breathing which could lead to a lot of diseases in latter life.

Gymnastics or aerobic exercises cannot be practiced by sick, weak and old person whereas in order to remove sickness, weakness and old age Yogasana can be practiced. In normal exercises one feels fatigue, tiredness and tensed but in Yogasana, one experiences lightness and relaxation. Other exercises increases the toxins in the body where as Yogasanas reduce the toxic levels. In Yogasana there is a very good co-ordination between the body, breath and mind. Exercises are limited to physical development whereas Yogasana develops not only the physical body but also a calm and steady mind, it also brings deep rhythmic breathing, free circulation of blood, vital and psychic energy and also awakening of the psychic centers, and thus leads us towards our goal of Self Realization.

Yogasanas and Health

So are Yogasanas different? Yes, they are completely different and far more comprehensive. As Yogasana is practiced slowly with relaxation and concentration, they influence both external and internal systems so that the nervous system, endocrine glands, internal organs and also the muscles are encouraged to function properly. Thus asanas have both physical and psychosomatic effect which is helpful in curing illness.

Physical Benefits

1) The endocrine system is one of the most important systems in our body. Asanas help to control and regulate the correct quantity of different hormones that are secreted from all the glands in the body. The endocrine glands in the physical body have their subtle replicas or representatives in the Mental body known as Chakras or energy centers. Hence the proper secretion of hormones has its own repercussions on physical as well as the psychological aspects of the practitioner. Therefore this system should be maintained at a peak condition.

2) By regular practice of asanas, diseased organs can be repaired, rejuvenated and put back to normalcy.

3) Asanas make the body flexible and able to adjust itself easily to climatic changes and also the environment.

4) It helps in proper digestion of food by stimulating correct amount of flow of the digestive juices like saliva, enzymes etc.

5) The sympathetic and parasympathetic systems are balanced so that the internal organs they control are neither hyperactive or hypoactive.

6) The muscles, the bones and all the systems of the body like nervous, glandular, respiratory, excretory and circulatory are coordinated so that they help each other.

7) Ailments associated with modern civilized life, such as constipation, rheumatism, stiffness, frustration and tension are released with the practice of asanas.

Hence by the regular practice of Yogasanas the physical body is maintained to the optimal level.

Mental Benefits

1) Stability of the mind is established and there is a release of dormant potentialities which makes it easy to face the difficulties of life.

2) By the regular practice of asanas; qualities such as determination, concentration, and self confidence are developed which are visible in the practitioner's speech behavior and actions.

3) Equipoise and vitality become the normal state of mind. You are able to face sorrows, anxieties and problems without being disturbed.

Spiritual Benefits

1) The practice of Asanas make the body steady and also purifies the body for higher techniques of Pratyahar (sense withdrawal), dharana (concentration) and dhyana (meditation) which ultimately leads to Samadhi (Cosmic realization).

2) Some people have the mistaken idea that asanas are for physical wellbeing and have no connection or use on the spiritual path. This is totally a wrong concept. The practice of asana may not give the direct experience of spiritual realization, but they are a stage on the eightfold path of Sai Asthang Yoga. They awaken the psychic faculties dormant in the spiritual aspirants.

3) All the meditative postures – Padmasana, Ardha Padmasana, Sukhasana etc. form 2 pyramids.

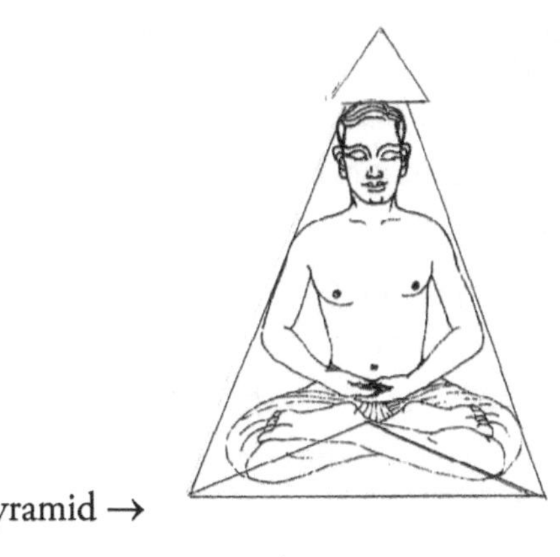

1st Pyramid →

↑ - 2nd Pyramid

These Pyramids give the following effects

1) In a pyramid the base has heat energy and the apex has cool energy.

2) When we sit in the above posture two different pyramids are formed, one at the top of the head, at the Sahasrara or crown chakra which gives the body and the mind the Prana or cosmic energy. Secondly, another pyramid is formed at the base that is the Mooladhar or root chakra, taking the earth energy.

3) This heat energy at the base helps in the cleansing of Shushmna Nadi and the other subtle nadis and also helps to awaken the Kindalini Shakti after a prolonged practice.

4) There is friction between the cool energy coming down from the apex and heat energy coming up from the base. This friction between the two energies creates electrifying effect on the spine which is very helpful in advance stages of meditation.

Thus, the practice of these postures helps us for proper assimilation, digestion and elimination processes in the body which are mainly at the lower part of the body and also keeps our mind and calm and peaceful at the upper part of the body that is our head.

Instructions to Be Followed Before Commencement of Practice of Asanas

The instructions, advice and precautions given below should be carefully studied before commencing the practice of asanas.

1) **Empty stomach:** The stomach should be empty while doing asanas. Early morning or 3 to 4 hours after lunch is advisable.

2) **Emptying of bowls:** Before starting the practice of asanas, the bladder and intestines should be preferably empty. Drinking two or three glasses of slightly salted water will facilitate the loosening of the bowels.

3) **Breathing:** always breathe through the nose, unless specific contrary instructions are given. Try to coordinate the respiration with the asana practice.

4) **Place of Practice:** Practice Yogasanas in a well-ventilated room with a calm and quiet atmosphere. The air in the room should be fresh so that there is free flow of oxygen for us to breathe. We can practice outdoors in an open beautiful garden with a lot of greenery's around. Do not practice in a strong wind, in the cold or in air that is dirty, smoky or which smells. Do not practice under an electric fan.

5) **Blanket:** Use a folded blanket or a thick mat for our practice. Do not use a mattress which is spongy or filled with air.

6) **Time of Practice:** Asanas can be practiced any time of the day, except after meals. The best time to practice is early morning when the stomach is empty, the atmosphere is pure, quiet and filled with solar radiations and the mind is calm. The practitioner may find that the muscles are most stiff at this time of the day compared to late afternoon when they become suppler.

7) **Clothes:** Loose, light and comfortable clothing should be used and remove spectacles, wristwatches and ornaments from our body before practicing the asanas.

8) **Bathing:** Try taking a cold shower before starting. This will greatly improve the effect of the asanas.

9) **Diet:** There are no special dietary rules for practitioners of asanas but it is better to eat natural food in reasonable moderation. The practitioner is advised to fill half his stomach with food, one quarter with water and to leave the remaining quarter empty. Food should be had to satisfy the hunger and not so much that we feel heavy and lazy. Eat to live rather than live to eat. If the aim of doing asanas is spiritual then we must avoid acidic and gastric food so that we do not suffer from acidity and gastric problems. If a person is suffering from a particular disease then dietary restriction should be imposed.

10) **Strain:** No undue strain and force should be exerted while practicing asanas. The beginners may find their muscles stiff but after the practice of several weeks they will find their muscles suppler.

11) **Age Limit:** Asanas can be practiced by people of all age groups, male and female.

12) **Restrictions:** People suffering from chronic diseases like ulcers, T.B., hernia or high or low blood pressure, cardiac problems or people with

fractured bones, spondylosis etc should consult a yoga teacher before commencing asanas.

13) **Awareness of the Body:** The practice of asanas should be done slowly with full awareness of the body. If there is a feeling of pain or pleasure, do not react to it but be aware of the feeling. This will help us to develop the powers of concentration and endurance.

14) **Relaxation:** Practice Shavasana before, during and after asana sessions, taking care to relax the body as much as possible. Though Shavasana looks easy, to relax completely is difficult.

15) **Termination of Asana:** If one experiences excessive pain in any part of the body, the asanas should be immediately terminated; if necessary, seek advice. Do not stay in an asana if excessive discomfort is felt.

16) **Inverted Asanas:** Do not practice inverted asanas if there is gas or fermentation in the intestines or if the blood is excessively impure. This is important to ensure that toxins do not go to the brain and cause damage.

PREPARATORY OR FREE –HAND SERIES OF EXERCISE

Before the actual practice of Asanas one should practice the Free-Hand series of exercises. They help to open up the joints, reactivate and stabilize the nerves and muscles of the body. Though they are very simple practices they lubricate the joints and make them more flexible. They stretch and strengthen the muscles and nerves and make them suppler. They relieve muscle cramps and strain on the joints. They establish free flow of Pranic or vital energy in the different parts of the body. They relieve stiffness and muscular tension and improve blood circulation in all the parts of the body. The hectic life schedule of modern man makes the functions of the different limbs and joints weak and prevents them from proper functioning. The old, the weak and people suffering from psychosomatic diseases and who are unable to do advance yogic practices can perform these more simple practices. In this way they can manage to overcome the weakness and regain the free movement of the whole body.

As per Ayurveda, an ancient medical science, there are three major aspects which exist in the body. They are known as Vata (wind), Pitta (acid or bile) and Kapha (phlegm or mucus). When these three factors are not balanced, the body malfunctions which causes diseases to occur. The Free Hand exercises can reestablish the balance.

Given below are the some of the few, Free Hand exercises which should be practiced regularly before starting the actual Asanas to loosen the muscles and joints of the body.

Before starting the Preparatory Free Hand exercises we must start with **Shavasana** (refer Relaxation postures) to relax physically and mentally.

Free Hand Exercises of Lower Extremities-legs.

Toe Bending and Ankle Bending:

Take the sitting position, with legs stretched out in front of the body (the basic posture) and hands at the sides. Lean backward taking support on the straight arms. Become aware of the toes and move the toes of both feet slowly backward and forward, keeping the feet rigid. Repeat 10 times.

Sit in the same position as above and move both feet backward and forward as much as possible, bending them from the ankle joints. Repeat 10 times.

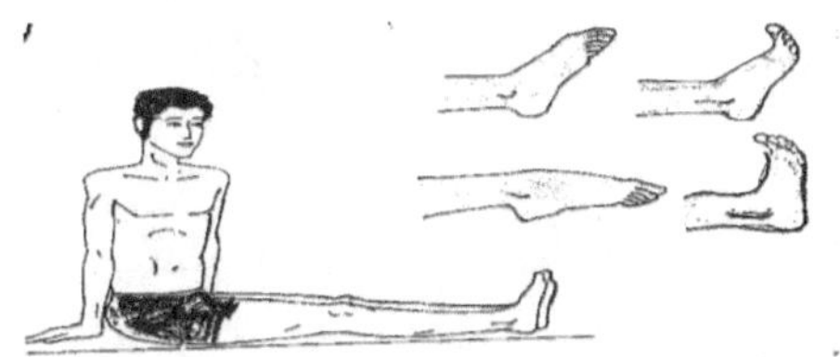

Ankle Rotation:

Sit in the same position as above. Separate the legs, keeping them Straight. Keep the heels in contact with the floor. Rotate the right foot from the ankle; clockwise 10 times and anticlockwise 10 times..

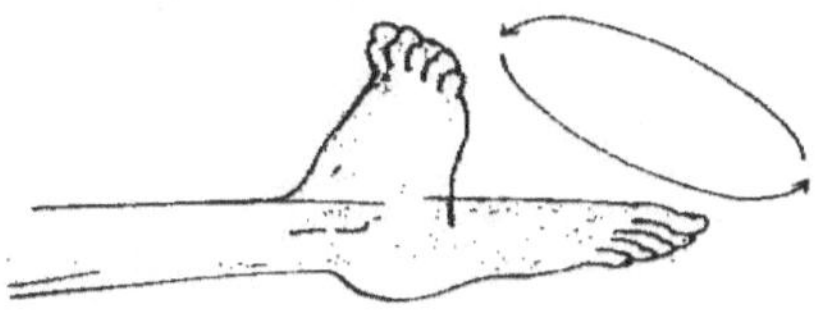

Repeat the same procedure with the left foot. Then rotate both feet together.

Knee Rotation:

Fold the right leg and place the right foot on the left thigh. Hold the right foot with the left hand. Rotate the right knee in a circle, trying to gradually make the circle larger. Repeat 10 times clockwise and 10 times anticlockwise. Repeat the same procedure with the left knee.

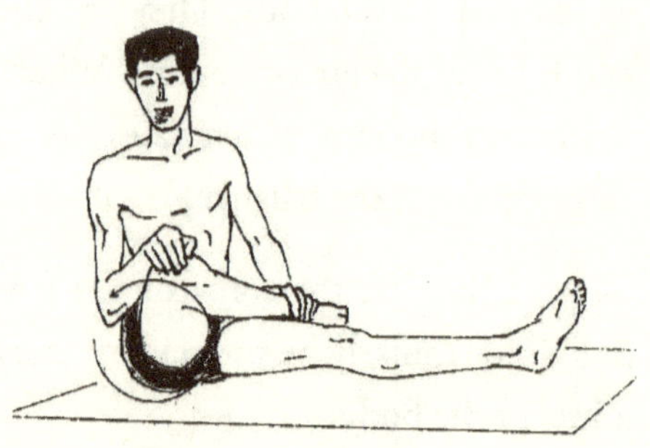

Half Butterfly:

Fold the right leg and place the right foot on the left thigh. Place the left hand on the right foot and the right hand on the top of the bent right knee. Gently move the bend leg up and down with the right hand allowing the muscles of the leg to relax as much as possible. Repeat the same process with the left knee. After some days or weeks of practice the knee should comfortably rest on the floor without effort.

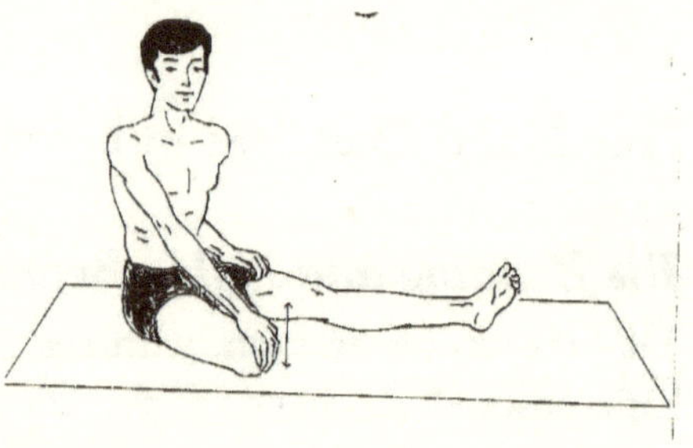

Full Butterfly:

Take a sitting position, bringing the soles of the feet together. Try to bring the heels as close to the body as possible. Place the hands on the knees. Utilizing the arms, push the knees towards the ground, allowing them to bounce upward again. Repeat this 20 to 25 times.

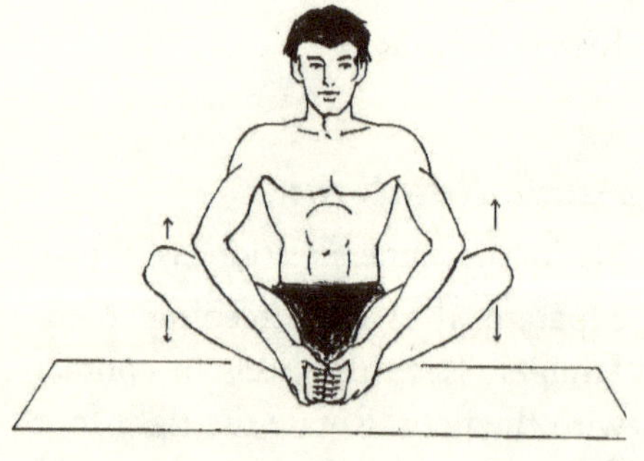

The same exercise can be done by holding the feet with clasped hands to keep them in the same position and then push the knees towards the ground.

Kagasana and Crow walking:

Take the position by squatting on the floor. Place the palms of the hands on the knees and begin to walk in the squatting position. One can walk either on the toes or the feet; choose whichever is most difficult. Practice this exercise for a short time without strain. Crow walk touching the knee to the ground with each step.

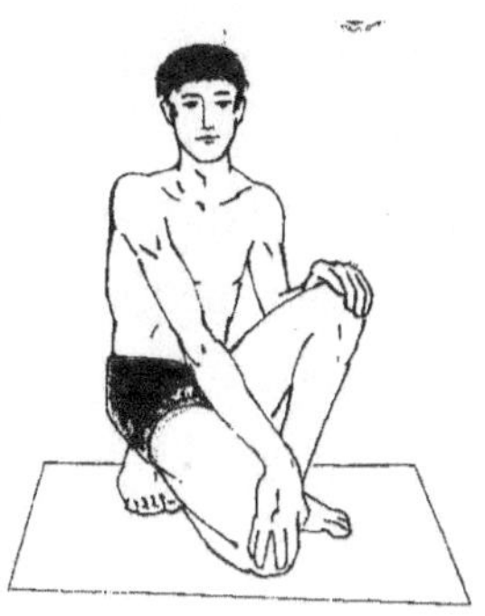

Benefits:

1) Helps to improve the circulation of blood in the legs.

2) This exercise is good for people suffering from constipation. They should drink 2 glasses of water and then crow walk for one minute. Drink 2 more glasses of water and crow walk again. Repeat 3 to 4 times; this will remove the constipation.

3) This is a very good exercise to prepare the legs for meditative postures.

Free Hand Exercises for Upper Extremities-hands.

Hand Clenching:

Hold the arms straight out in front of the body, so that they are on the same horizontal plane as the shoulders.

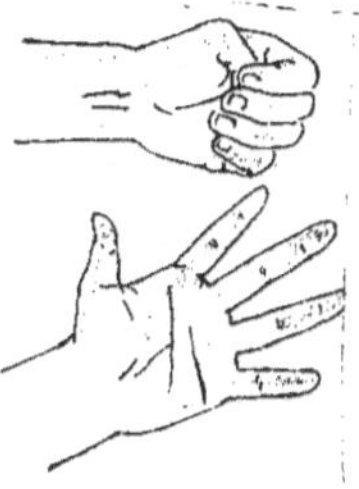

Stretch and tense the fingers of both hands and then close the fingers over the thumb to make a tight fist. Again stretch and tense the fingers. Repeat this movement 10 times.

Wrist Bending:

Maintain the same position of the hands as above. Bend the hands at the wrist as if we are pressing the palms against a wall, with the fingers pointing upwards. Then again bend the hands at the wrist and point the fingers downwards. Again point the fingers upwards. Repeat 10 times.

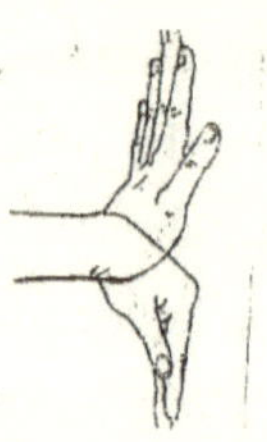

Wrist Joint Rotation:

Hold the right hand straight in front of the body, so that it is on the same horizontal plane as the shoulder. Clench the right fist and rotate it clockwise 10 times from the wrist and then rotate it anticlockwise 10 times. Repeat the same movement with the left hand. Extend both arms in front of the body with the fists clenched. Now rotate the fists together 10 times clockwise and 10 times anticlockwise.

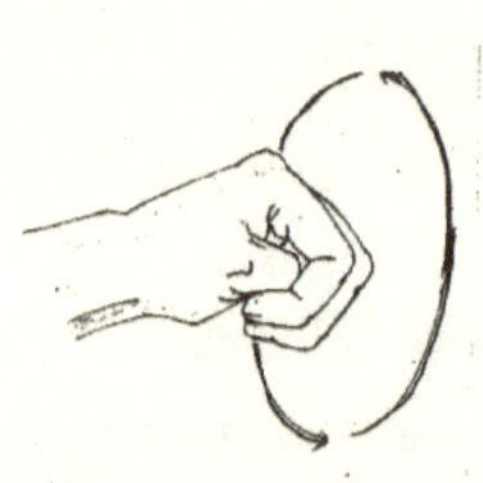

Elbow Bending:

a) Hold both the arms outstretched with the hands open and palms uppermost. Bend both the arms at the elbows, touch the shoulders with the fingers, then straighten the arms again. Repeat 10 times.

b) Perform the same exercise but with the arms extended sideways. Repeat 10 times.

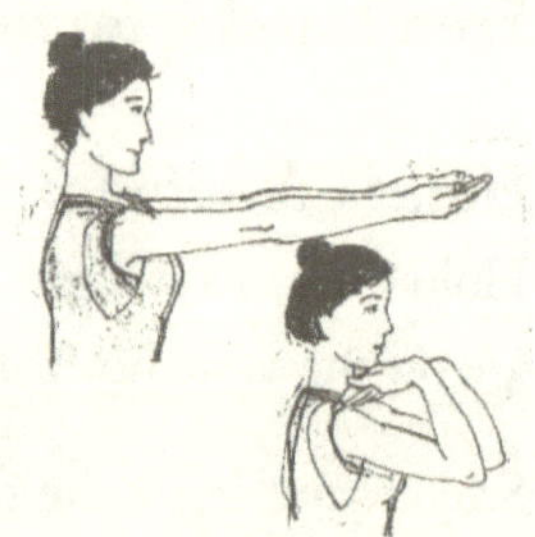

Shoulder Rotation:

Take the same position as mentioned in the above exercise. Make a circular movement from the shoulder joints; keeping the fingers in contact with the shoulders. Do it 10 times clockwise and 10 times anticlockwise. Try to make the circular movement of each elbow as large as possible, bringing the two elbows in contact with each other in front of the chest.

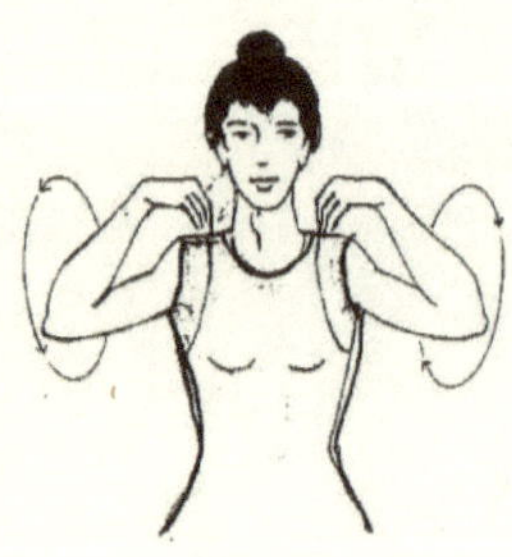

Neck Movements:

These exercises can be done in sitting or standing position.

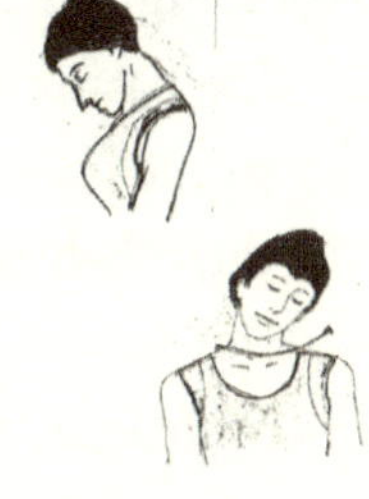

a) Slowly move the head backward and forward 10 times.

b) Slowly tilt the head to the right and then to the left, first while facing directly forward and then while turning the head to the left and right. Repeat both the methods 10 times each.

c) Slowly rotate the head in as large a circle as possible 10 times clockwise and 10 times anticlockwise, without jerking or straining.

Benefits: All the nerves connecting the different parts of the body with the brain must pass through the neck. This vital passage is exercised and toned by the above movements.

Cycling:

a) Take a sleeping position with the back flat on the ground. Raise the right leg and make 10 forward cycling movements followed by 10 reverse cycling movements. Repeat the same procedure with the left leg.

b) Using both legs make alternate cycling movements, 10 times forward and then 10 times in reverse.

c) Now keep the legs locked together and do 10 forward and 10 reverse cycling movements.

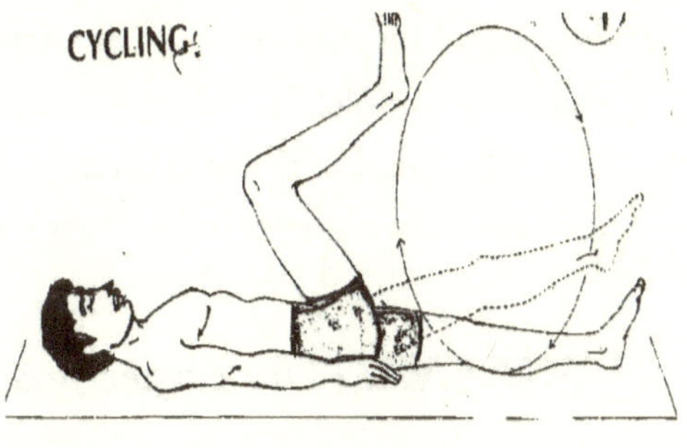

Note: After completion of this exercise, rest, lying flat on the back until respiration returns to normal. Do not strain.

Rocking and Rolling:

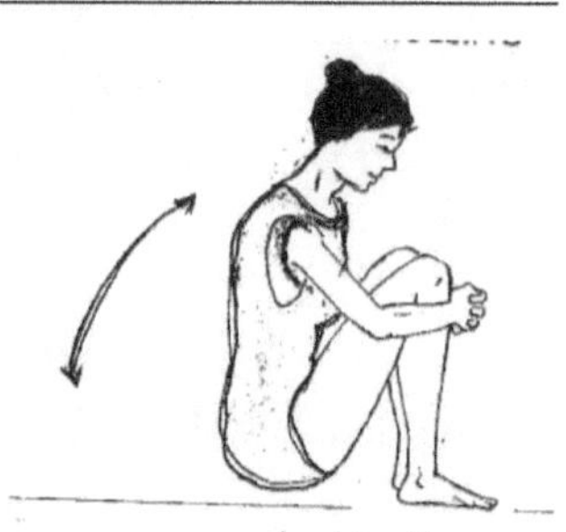

a) Lie flat on the back. Fold both the legs up to the chest. Interlock the fingers and place them behind the head. Roll the body from side to side, keeping the elbows on the floor.

b) Remain in the same position; wrap the arms around the knees and rock the whole body along the spinal cord. Try to come on the squatting position on the feet.

Note: Use a folded blanket for this practice so that no damage is done to the spine. Be careful that the head does not hit the ground with force.

Limitations: Not to be done by persons with spinal problems. **Benefits:** This exercise is most beneficial if done just after awakening in the morning. This exercise massages the back, buttocks and hips.

Relaxation Postures Series

The Benefits of Relaxation Postures are:

a) It is useful for those people who have trouble even during sleep. It relaxes the body completely and gives the body rest that it badly needs.

b) They should be performed directly before starting the asana session and at any time when the body becomes tired.

SHAVASANA: (The corpse pose)

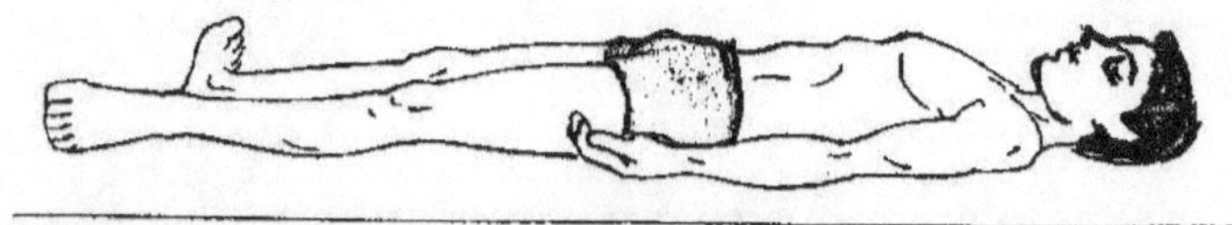

Lie flat on the back with the arms at the sides and in line with the body, palms facing upward. Close the eyes and keep the feet slightly apart. Relax the body completely from head to toe. Concentrate on the breath till the breath becomes rhythmic and natural. Continue concentrating on the inhalation and exhalation. If the mind wanders bring it back to the breath. If you can keep the mind on the breath for a few minutes, the mind and body will relax.

Duration: In general, the longer we do this, the better it is, but during asana practice a minute or two is sufficient.

Benefits: It relaxes the entire psychological system. Shavasana is practiced before sleep, or during asana practice and after dynamic exercises such as Surya namaskara.

ADVASANA: (the reversed corpse pose)

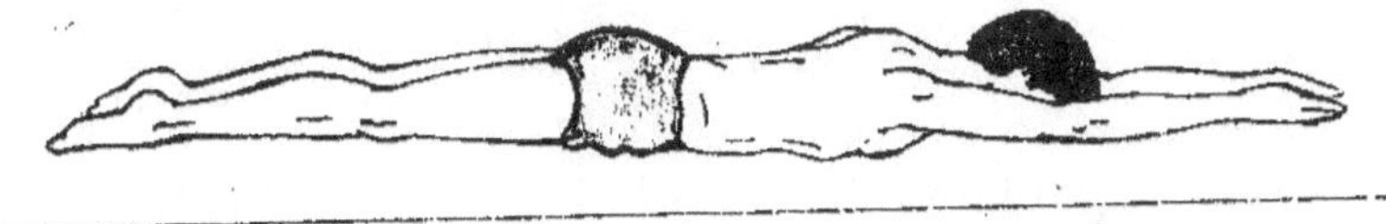

Lie on the stomach. Stretch arms forward on each side of the head. Relax the whole body in the same way as described above in Shavasana.

Breath: Breathing should be natural, normal and rhythmic.

Duration: This asana should be practiced as long as possible if it is for a specific treatment. A few minutes of practice is sufficient, before or during the asana practice.

Benefits: This posture is recommended for people suffering from slipped disc, stiff neck and stooping figure. They will find this posture an excellent sleeping pose.

MAKARASANA: (The Crocodile pose)

Lie flat on the stomach. Raise the head and shoulders and rest the head in the palms of the hands with the elbows on the ground. Close the eyes and relax the whole body.

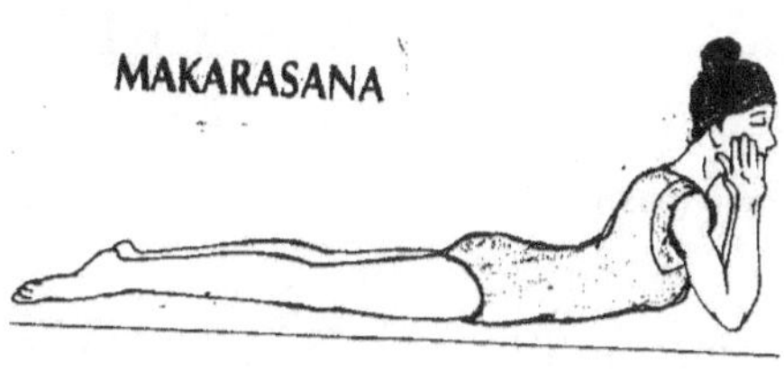

Breath: Breathing should be normal, natural and rhythmic.

Duration: Lie in this position till we are comfortable, as long as possible.

Benefits: People suffering from any lung ailments or asthma should practice this simple asana. This asana is very effective for persons suffering from slipped disc or any spinal disorder. They should practice this asana for extended period of time.

MATSYA KRIDASANA: (The flapping fish pose).

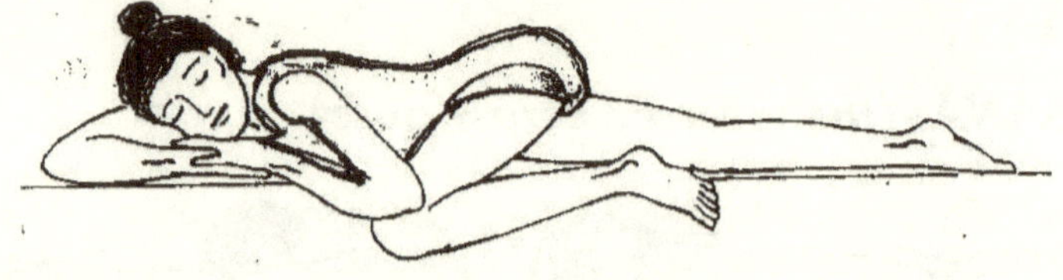

Lie on the stomach with the fingers interlocked under the head. Fold the left leg sideways and bring the left knee close to the ribs. Swivel the arms to the left and rest the left elbow on the left knee. Rest the right side of the head on the crook of the right arm. This position resembles a flapping fish.

Breath: Breathing should be normal, relaxed in the static pose.

Duration: This asana should be practiced as much as possible on both the sides and can be used for sleeping.

Benefits: This asana redistributes waistline fat deposits and stimulates digestive peristalsis by stretching the intestines and helps remove constipation. The sciatic pain is relieved because this asana relaxes the nerves in the legs. It is an excellent resting pose.

MEDITATIVE POSTURES SERIES

The importance of meditative posture is to allow the practitioner to sit in one position with spine erect for an extended period of time, in the advanced stages of meditation. This helps the person to meditate successfully. The asanas in this series can be maintained for a long time without strain and discomfort. In higher stages of meditation, the practitioner loses control over the muscles of the body and it is at that time, these asanas are helpful to automatically hold the body in a steady position.

Beginners may start with Sukhasana and later prepare the body for other meditative poses like Padmasana or Siddhasana.

Precautions: If there is severe pain in the legs after some time in a meditative asana, slowly unlock the legs and massage them and then again sit in the asana. Do not strain or use undue force to sit in the asana.

PADMASANA: (the lotus pose)

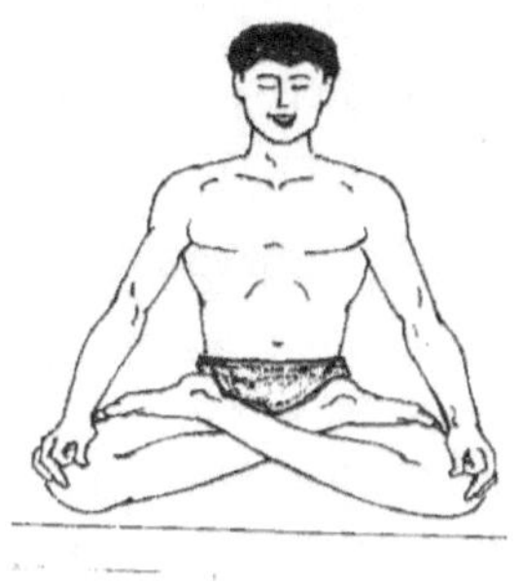

Sit with the legs extended forward. Fold one leg and place its foot on the top of the opposite thigh. The sole of the foot must be upward and the heel should touch the pelvic bone. Fold the other leg and place its foot on top of the other thigh.

Note: Beginners may find it easy to maintain this posture if they place a low cushion under their buttocks before assuming the pose.

While practicing this Posture we can also practice gyana mudra or chin mudra (refer to 'Hasta Mudras' for details). The spine must be steady and completely upright as though it is fixed to the ground.

Limitations: This posture **should not** be practiced by persons with sciatica or sacral infections. **Precautions:** One should not attempt this asana unless the person has developed supple legs after the practicing of the Preparatory exercises like crow walking, half and full butterfly etc.

Benefits:

1) When this posture is mastered, the practitioner is able to hold his body completely steady for long periods of time.
2) As the body and mind are interlinked and control each other, the steadiness of the body brings the steadiness of the mind and is the first step towards productive meditation.

3) The proper flow of Prana is directed from the Muladhar chakra (in the perineum) to the Sahasrara (in the head).

4) Padmasana tones the coccygeal and sacral nerves by supplying them with an extra flow of blood. It also helps to clear up many physical, nervous and emotional problems.

5) It also stimulates the digestive system.

ARDHA PADMASANA: (Half lotus pose)

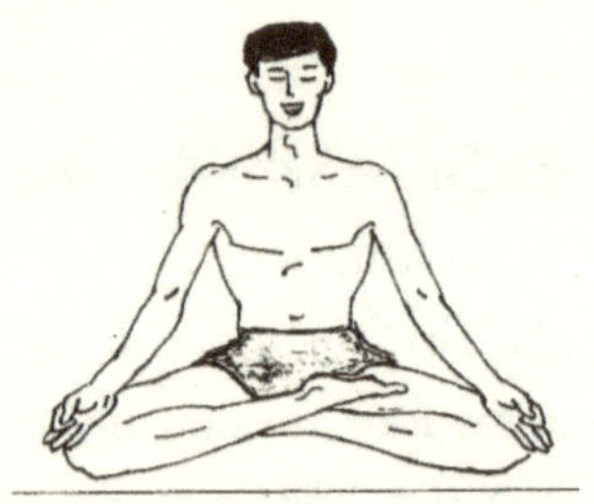

Sit with the feet stretched in front of the body. Fold the left leg and place the left foot beside the right thigh. Fold the right leg and place the right foot on the top of the left thigh. Keep the back, neck and head straight.

This pose is to be practiced in preference to sukhasana. By practicing this asana by using alternate leg positions, the practitioner will slowly prepare for Padmasana.

Limitations and Benefits: Same as padmasana but with a reduced level.

SUKHASANA (the easy posture)

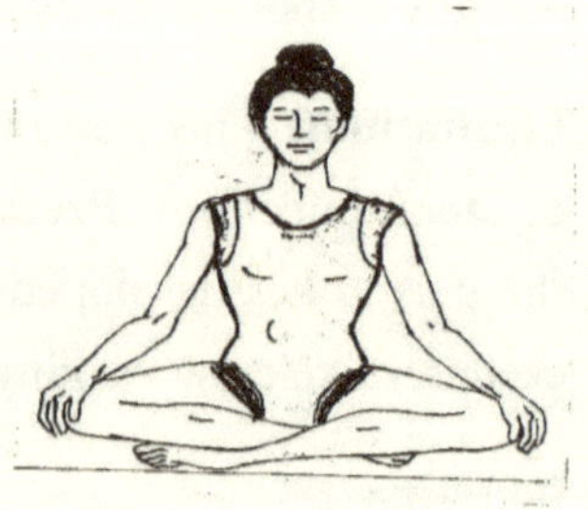

Sit with legs stretched in front of the body. Fold the right foot under the left thigh and fold the left foot under the right thigh. Place the hands of the knees and keep the head, neck and back straight.

This asana is for the beginners or for those who are not comfortable with other meditative poses.

VAJRASANA: (the thunderbolt pose)

Stand on the knees with the feet stretched backward and big toes crossed. The knees should be together, heels apart. Lower the buttocks onto the insides of the feet, the heels at the sides of the hips. Place the hands on the knees, palm downwards.

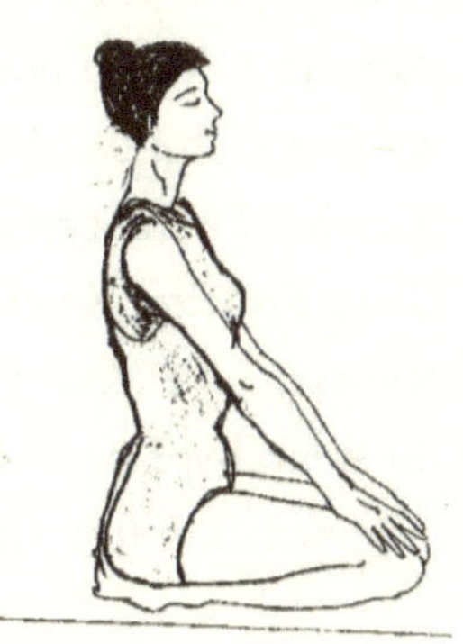

When this asana is practiced by concentrating on the normal breath with eyes closed, it brings tranquility to the mind.

Duration: Practice Vajrasana as much as possible, especially straight after meals for at least 5 minutes to enhance the digestive function.

Note: Vajrasana is the prayer pose of the Muslims and meditation pose of the Japanese Buddhists. **Benefits:** This pose enhances the efficiency of the entire digestive system, especially for persons suffering from indigestion. It strengthens the pelvic muscles which helps to prevent hernia and aids women in childbirth. It is useful in relieving stomach ailment such as peptic ulcers and hyperacidity.

SURYA NAMASKAR: (Salutations to the Sun)

This dynamic exercise is traditionally not regarded as part of Yoga practice. As it is a very good method of loosening up all the joints and muscles in the body as well as massaging all the internal organs and as it comprises 12 different asanas in itself, it has been included in this book. It is an excellent exercise to be done regularly early in the morning after bath or if one feels tired at any time of the day. This exercise restores lost vitality both physically and mentally.

One complete round of surya namasakar consists of 12 asanas performed in succession twice. Associated with each of the 12 positions is a mantra which should be chanted verbally or mentally for optimum benefit.

Positions from 1 to 12 constitute half round of Surya Namaskar. Second round, the positions are repeated but with a few minor changes.

PRANAMASANA: *(the prayer pose*

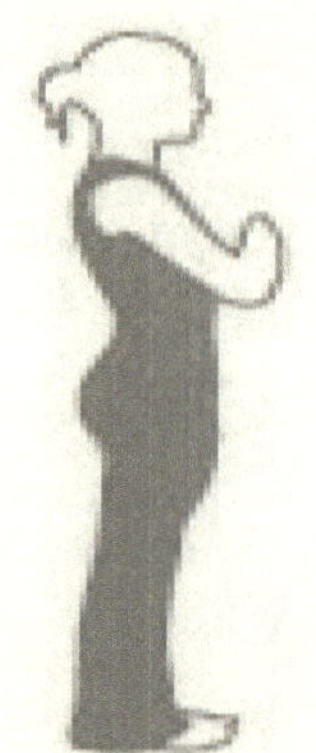

Position 1- Stand erect with the feet together. Place the palms together in front of the chest. Relax the whole body.

Breath: Normal breathing.

Concentration: On the Anahata or Heart Chakra

Mantra: Om Mitraya Namaha (Salutations to the friend of all) **Benefits:** Establishes a state of concentration and calmness in preparation for exercise to be done.

HASTA UTTANASANA: *(the raised arms pose)*

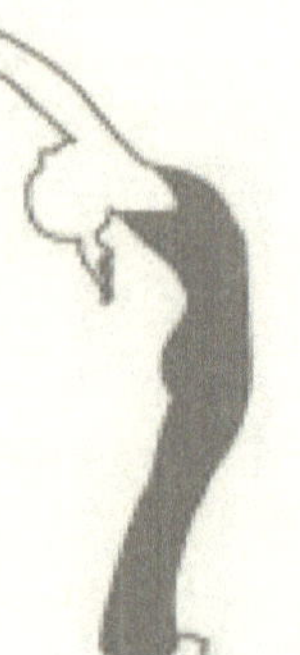

Position 2- Raise both arms above the head. Keep the arms separated by one shoulder's width. Bend the head and upper trunk backward.

Breath: Inhale while raising the arms.

Concentration: On Vishuddhi or throat chakra

Mantra: Om Ravaye Namaha (Salutation to the shining one) **Benefits:** Gives good exercise to the arm and shoulder muscles tones the spinal nerves, opens all the lung compartments, stretches the abdominal area and removes excess fat and improves digestion.

PADAHASTASANA: *(the hand to foot pose)*

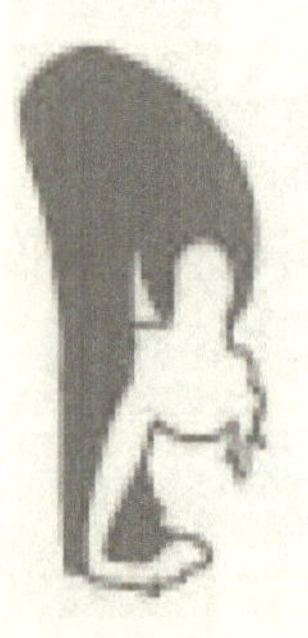

Position 3- Bend forward and let the palms and fingers touch the ground either on both sides of the feet or in front of the feet and try touching the knees with the forehead. Do not strain. Keep the legs straight.

Breath: Exhale while bending forward and contract the abdomen so that maximum amount of air is expelled.

Concentration: Swadhistana Chakra.

Mantra: Om Suryaya Namaha (Salutations to Him who induces activity).

Benefits: Removes surplus abdominal fats, improves digestion, removes constipation, improves blood circulation makes the spine supple and tones the spinal nerves, eliminates abdominal ailments.

ASHWA SANCHALANASANA: (the equestrian pose)

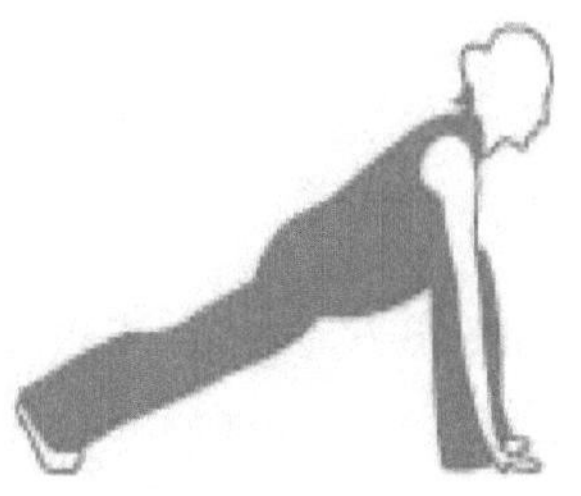

Position 4- First bend both the knees and place the palms flat on the floor on either side of the feet. Stretch the right leg back as far as possible but keep the left foot in the same position.

The arms should remain straight and in the same position. Overall the weight of the body should be supported on the two hands, the left foot, the right knee and the toes of the right foot. The head should be tilted backward, the back arched and the gaze directed upward.

Breath Inhale while stretching the right leg backward.

Concentration: Ajna Chakra

Mantra: Om Bhanave Namaha (Salutations to he who illumines)

Benefits: Nervous balance improves, the function of the abdominal organs improve and muscles of the legs are strengthened.

PARVATASAN: (the mountain pose)

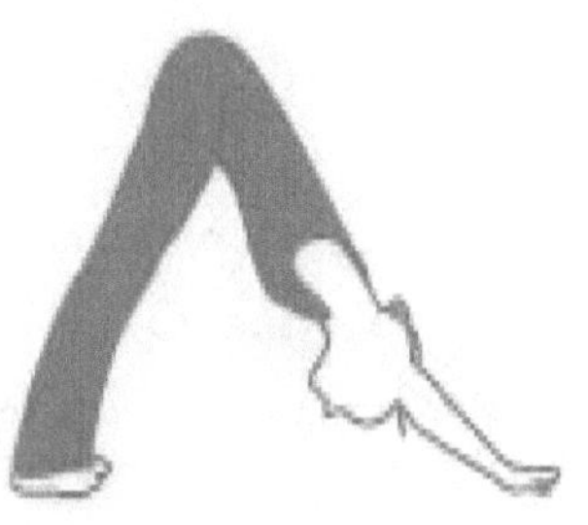

Position 5- Straighten the left leg and place the left foot besides the right foot. Raise the buttocks in the air and lower the head so that it lies between the two arms; the body should form two sides of a triangle. In the final position the legs and arms should be straight. In this pose; try to keep the heels in contact with the ground.

Breath: Exhale while straightening the left leg and bending the trunk.

Concentration: Vishuddhi chakra.

Mantra: Om Khagaya Namaha (Salutation to he who moves quickly in the sky)

Benefits: Tones the spinal nerves and makes the spine supple. Improves circulation of blood in the spinal area. Strengthens the muscles and nerves of arms and legs.

ASTANGANAMASKARA: (the salutation with 8 limbs)

Position 6- Lower the body to the ground so that in the final position, only the toes of both feet, the two knees, the chest, the hands and the chin touch the ground. The hips and the abdomen should be raised slightly off the ground.

Breath: The breath should be held outside. No respiration.

Concentration: On Manipur Chakra

Mantra: Om Pushne Namaha (Salutation to the giver of strength).

Benefits: Develops the chest and strengthens the muscles of arms and legs.

BHUJANGASANA: (the Cobra pose)

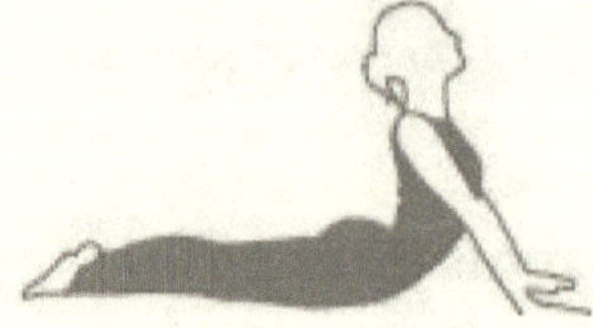

Position 7- Straighten the arms and lift the body from the waist. Bend the head backward. This final stage is the same as Bhujangasana.

Breath: Inhale while raising the body and stretching the back.

Concentration: On Swadhistana chakra

Mantra: Om Hiranya Garbhaya Namaha (Salutation to the golden cosmic self.)

Benefits: This pose is very useful for all stomach ailments, including indigestion and constipation, all spinal problems because, arching the back revitalizes the most important spinal nerves.

PARVATASAN: (the mountain pose)

Position 8- This stage is a repeat of position 5. From the arched back position assume the mountain pose as described in Posture 5.

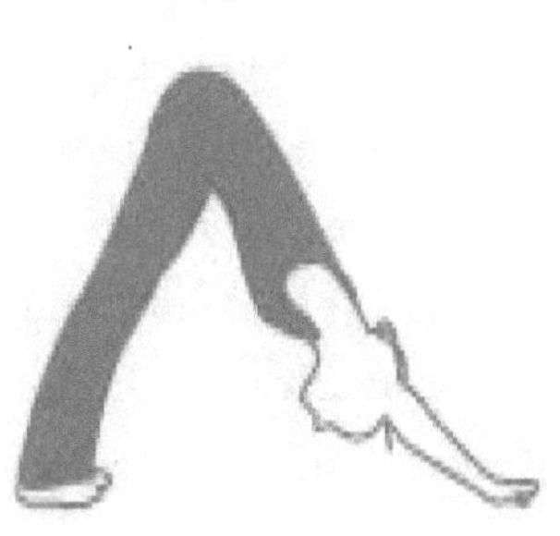

Breath: Exhale as you raise the buttocks.
Concentration: Vishuddhi chakra.
Mantra: Om Marichaye Namaha (Salutations to the lord of dawn).

ASHWA SANCHALANASANA: (the equestrian pose)

Position 9- This stage is the same as position 4. Bend the left leg and bring the left foot forward so that it lies near the hands. At the same time lower the right knee so that it touches the floor.

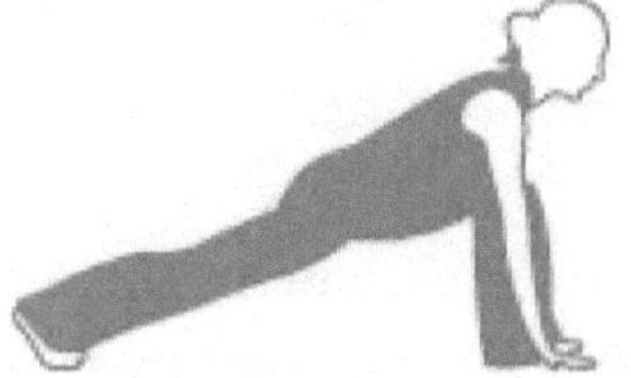

Breath: Inhale while assuming the pose.
Concentration: Ajna Chakra
Mantra: Om Adityaya Namaha (Salutation to the son of Aditi) Aditi is one of the names of the infinite cosmic mother.

PADAHASTASANA: (the hand to foot pose)

Position 10- This position is the repeat of position 3. Place the right foot next to the left foot. **Rest is same as position 3.**

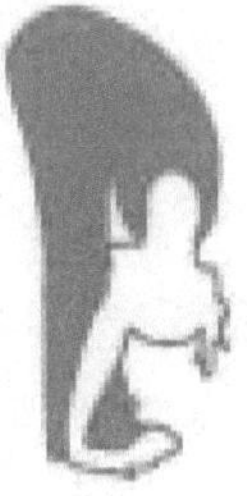

Breath: Exhale while performing the movement.
Concentration: Swadhistana chakra.
Mantra: Om Savitre Namaha (Salutations to the benevolent mother).

HASTA UTTANASANA: (the raised arms pose).

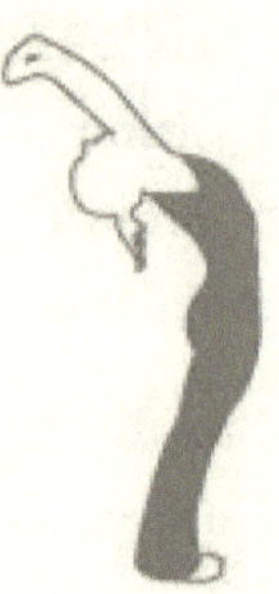

Position 11- This stage is the repeat of position 2. Straighten the whole body and raise the arms above the head. **Rest is same as position 2.**

Breath: Inhale while straightening the body.

Concentration: Vishuddhi chakra

Mantra: Om Arkaya Namaha (Salutations to he who is fit to be praised).

PRANAMASANA: (the prayer pose).

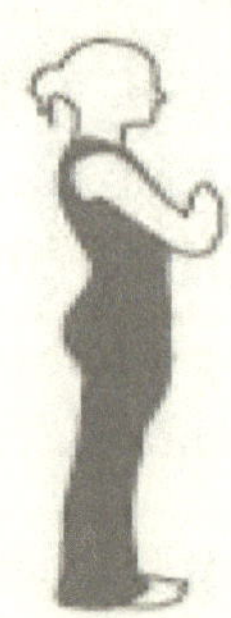

Position 12- This is the final pose and is the same as position 1. Bring the hands in front of the chest and place the palms together. Relax whole body.

Breath: Exhale while assuming the final pose

Concentration: Anahat chakra

Mantra: Om Bhaskaraya Namaha (Salutations to he who leads to enlightenment).

Positions 13 to 24

The positions 1 to 12 shown above constitute half a round of Surya Namaskara. For completion of 1 full round the second half, positions 1 to 12 are repeated with a few minor changes, by exchange of the leg positions.

For example, in position 4, instead of stretching the right foot backward, stretch the left foot back in the same way. And in position 9 bend the right leg and bring the right foot near the hands.

DURATION: If Surya Namaskar is practiced for spiritual benefit, then practice 3 to 12 rounds slowly. For physical benefits, practice 3 to 12 rounds more quickly. Beginners should not do a large number of rounds. They should start with 2 to 3 and then subsequently add one more.

After the practice of Surya namaskar the practitioner is advised to do Shavasana for a few minutes to allow the heart beat and respiration to return to normal, and to relax all the muscles in the body.

PRECAUTIONS: If the practitioner develops fever, then the practice of Surya Namaskara should be immediately discontinued. This happens due to toxins in the body. These toxins should be eliminated by practicing other asanas for a period of time and then Surya Namaskara can again be commenced.

LIMITATIONS: There are no age limits regarding the practice of Surya Namaskara; both young and old can practice it. Ladies however should not do this practice after the fourth month of pregnancy.

GENERAL BENEFITS: As a result of the whole practice, Surya Namaskar has a very powerful influence on all the systems of the body, endocrine, circulatory, digestive respiratory, muscular, nervous etc. and helps to bring them to balance with each other.

Daily practice of this exercise removes excessive fat and revitalizes the body and mind and sharpens the thinking faculty. Impurities are eliminated from the body in the form of perspiration. Breathing improves, which brings about oxygen-enriched air, providing oxidized blood to the brain, which in turn increases mental clarity. Thus, it bestows good physical and mental health to one and all.

Chandra Namaskar

The word 'chandra' means moon and the word namaskara means salutations. The waxing and the wanning moon have tremendous effect on the mind – the human behavior, the nature and seasons.

The 'Sukla Paksha';known as the bright fortnight from new moon to full moon, is the waxing moon and 'Krishna Paksha' known as the dark fortnight is when the moon. wanes to no moon. These processes take 15 days each. In accordance with this there are 15 body movements to maintain the balance between the body and the mind which are known as 'Chandra Namaskar'.

The difference between Surya Namaskar and Chandra Namaskar is:

a) In Surya Namaskar the Pingala nadi gets activated more, whereas in Chandra Namaskar the Ida nadi gets activated more.

b) Practice of Surya Namaskar gives a lot of heat, energy, strength and flexibility, whereas Chandra Namaskar develops a calm and cool mind.

(For details of Ida and Pingala Nadi's, please refer Chapter on Pranayama)

The ideal time to practice Chandra Namaskar is in the afternoon or at dusk. One can also do it in the morning. Preferably Surya Namaskar should be practiced in the morning and Chandra Namaskar in the evening.

PRANAMASANA: (Salutation in lightning bolt pose)

Position 1 – Sit in Vajrasana (see page 135) and join the palms in front of the chest in a relaxed salutation pose.

Breath: Breathe normally. **Concentration:** Anahat or heart chakra. **Benefits:** Same as Vajrasana.

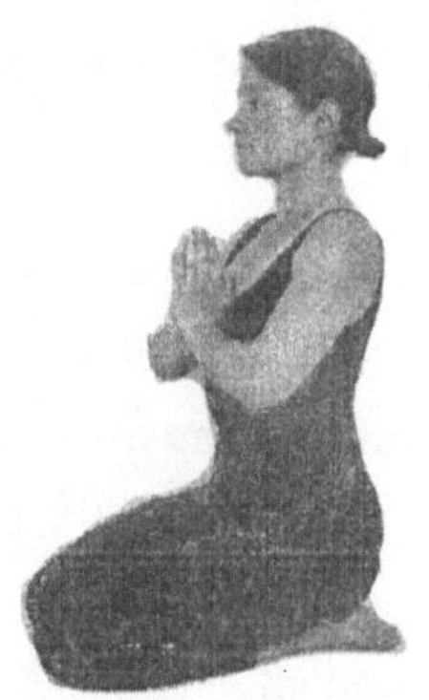

UTTHAN PRANAMASANA:
(Raised arms salutation pose)

Position 2 – From position 1, without separating the palms raise the hands over the shoulders and arch the back while inhaling.
Breath: Inhale slowly while raising the arms.
Concentration: Vishuddhi or throat chakra.
Benefits: Same as Hasta Utthanasana (refer to Surya Namaskar)

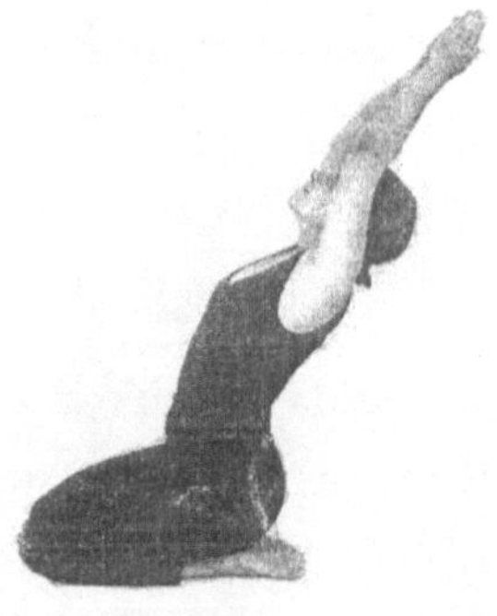

SHASANKASANA: *(moon pose)*

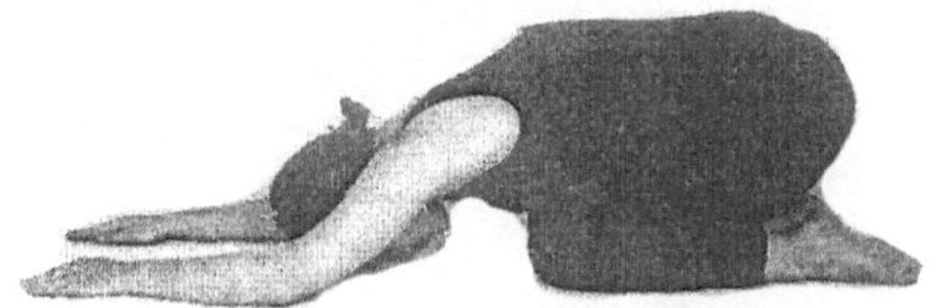

Position 3 – From position 2 Exhale slowly while bending forward from the hip joint. Keep the arms aligned with the trunk while bending forward. Place the forehead and arms on the floor with palms facing downwards.

Breath: Exhale slowly while bending forward.

Concentration: Manipur or navel chakra.

Benefits: Relieves tension, has soothing effect on the mind, develops concentration, regulates digestion, tones the pelvic muscles, removes constipation and gas, effective pose for hernia, asthma and diabetes.

BHUJANGASANA: *(Cobra Pose)*

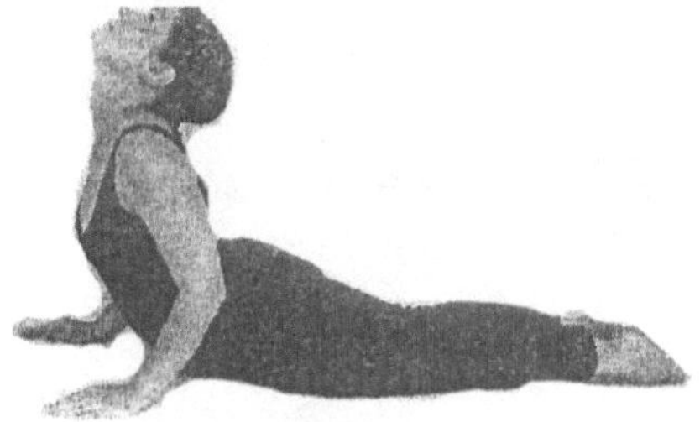

Position 4 – From position 3, straighten the arms and lift the body from the waist. Bend the head backward. This final stage is the same as Bhujangasana.

Breath: Inhale slowly while lifting the body.

Concentration: Manipur or navel chakra.

Benefits: same as Bhujangasana (refer to Surya Namaskar)

PARVATASAN: *(Mountain pose)*

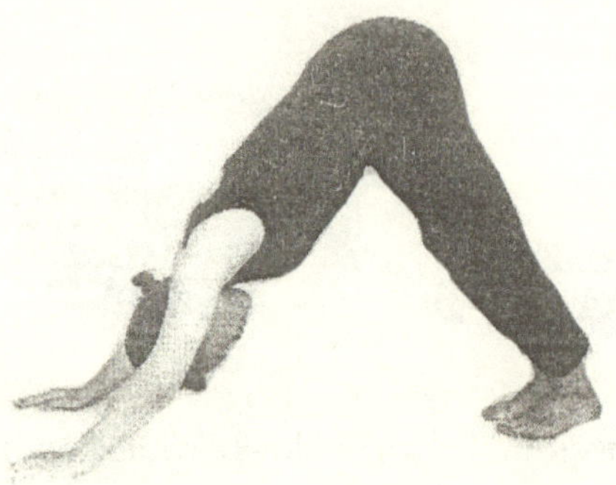

Position 5 – Continuing from position 4, Raise the buttocks in the air and lower the head so that it lies between the two arms; the body should form two sides of a triangle. In the final position the legs and arms should be straight. In this pose; try to keep the heels in contact with the ground.

Breath: Exhale while raising the buttocks.

Concentration: Vishuddhi chakra.

Benefits: Tones the Spinal nerves and makes the spine supple. Improves circulation of blood in the spinal area. Strengthens the muscles and nerves of arms and legs.

ARDHA CHANDRASANA: *(Half moon pose)*

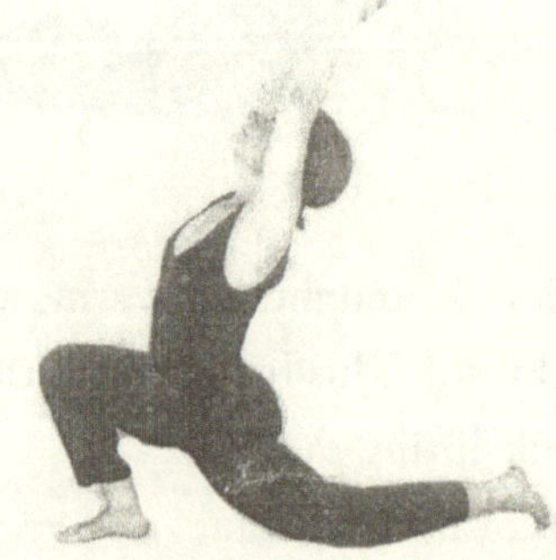

Position 6 – Continuing from position 5, move the right foot forward and raise the arms over the head and join the palms together. Arch the back and stretch the arms backwards.

Breath: Inhale, stretching the right leg forward **Concentration:** Ajna Chakra

Benefits: Nervous balance improves, the function of the abdominal organs improve and muscles of the legs are Strengthened.

PADAHASTASANA: (Feet and hand pose)

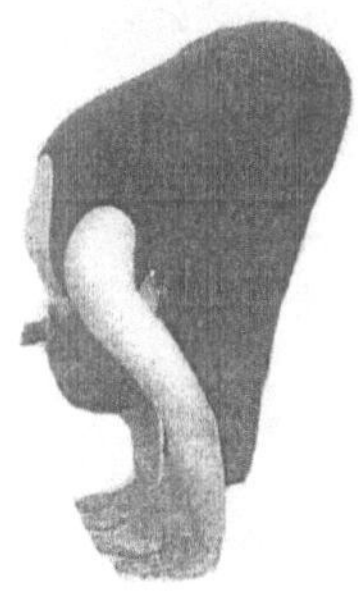

Position 7 – Bring the left foot from behind and join the right foot. Bend forward and let the palms and fingers touch the ground either on both sides of the feet or in front of the feet. Try touching the knees with the forehead. Do not strain. Keep the legs straight.

Breath: Exhale while bending forward and contract the abdomen so that maximum of air is expelled.

Concentration: Swadhistana Chakra.

Benefits: Removes surplus abdominal fat, improves digestion, removes constipation, improves blood circulation, makes the spine supple and tones the spinal nerves, eliminates abdominal ailments.

HASTA UTTHANASAN: (raised arm pose)

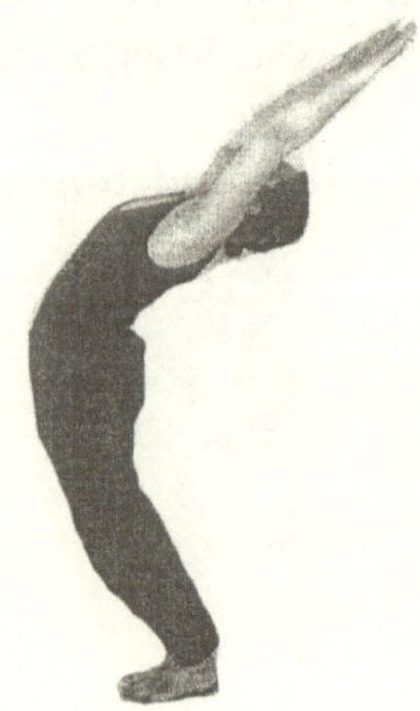

Position 8 – Raise the arms along with the upper body. Raise both arms above the head. Keep the arms separated by one shoulder's width. Bend the head and upper trunk backward.

Breath: Inhale while raising the arms.

Concentration: On Mooladhar or root chakra

Benefits: Gives good exercise to the arm and shoulder muscles tones the spinal nerves, opens all the lung compartments, stretches the abdominal area and removes excess fat and improves digestion.

Positions 9 to 15

Positions 9 to 15 are repetition as follows:

- Position 9 is same as Position 7
- Position 10 is same as Position 6
- Position 11 is same as Position 5
- Position 12 is same as Position 4
- Position 13 is same as Position 3
- Position 14 is same as Position 2
- Position 15 is same as Position 1

Complete Round of Chandra Namaskara:

The above stated 15 rounds constitute half the round of Chandra Namaskar placing the left leg to the rear in practice 6 to 10. The only change will be to place the right leg in the rear and complete the next 15 rounds. Therefore one round of Chandra Namaskar covers 30 movements.

DURATION: For people with normal health 5 to 6 rounds of Chandra Namaskar is sufficient for one day. All those who have time can practice 10 to 15 rounds.

Relax for 2 to 3 minutes in Shavasana after Chandra Namaskar. Always perform the exercise slowly and smoothly.

PRECAUTIONS: People suffering from high blood pressure, heart disease and pregnant ladies should not perform the practice of Chandra namaskara.

GENERAL BENEFITS: As a result of the whole practice, Chandra Namaskar has a very powerful influence on all the systems of the body, endocrine, circulatory, digestive respiratory, muscular, nervous etc. and helps to bring them to balance with each other.

Daily practice of this exercise removes excessive fat and revitalizes the body and mind and sharpens the thinking faculty. Impurities are eliminated from the body in the form of perspiration. Breathing improves, which brings about oxygen enriched air, which providing oxidized blood to the brain, which increases the mental clarity. Thus it bestows good physical and mental health to one and all. Chandra Nadi or Ida (left nostril) is activated which brings clarity of thought, concentration and keeps the mind cool and calm.

After the study of the important Asanas, let us now see what 'Bandha' means. Bandha or contractions are important part of Sai Ashtang Yoga and can be practiced individually and also while practicing Pranayama.

(Chandra Namaskar, Source:- 'Steps to Raja Yoga' by Swami Atmatattwananda Saraswati)

BANDHA
What is a Bandha?

Bandha means 'to hold or to tighten or to contract'. By the practice of these techniques; various parts of the body are gently but powerfully contracted and tightened. Practicing of bandha helps in removal of stagnant blood and stimulates and regulates the nerves connected with the organs. Overall it improves the functioning and keeps the body healthy, fit and fine.

These Bandha's also have a subtle effect on the chakras or energy centers which help the free flow of Prana in the Astral or Mental body especially the Susumna Nadi. They also help in the spiritual growth of the practitioner.

These bandhs can be practiced all by themselves or together with Pranayama and or Mudras (which are described in the next Chapter of Pranayama).

JALANDER BANDHA (the chin lock)

This bandh can be practiced in sitting as well as standing position. Sit comfortable in a meditative posture, where the knees can firmly touch the floor. Close the eyes and relax the body. Place the palms on the knees. Inhale slowly and deeply and retain the breath inside, bend the head a little forward. Hunch the shoulder upward and forward and press the chin tightly against the chest (near the sternum). See that the hands are straight and firmly set in position to hold the torso in position.

Stay in this position as long as we are comfortably able to retain the breath and concentrate on the Vishudha Chakra.

Then slowly relax the shoulder, bend the arms, release the lock by raising the head and exhale. Repeat the process when the respiration is normal. The same practice can be performed with the breath retained outside.

Duration: Repeat the exercise 10 times or as long as we can hold the breath comfortably.

Caution: Never inhale or exhale when the Bandha is on or in progress. People suffering from heart ailments or high blood pressure should not perform this exercise without proper guidance.

Benefits: The thyroid and the parathyroid glands are massaged and their function is improved. Relieves stress, anxiety, anger and brings tranquility to the mind.

UDDIYANA BANDHA (the abdominal lock)

This bandha can be practiced in sitting as well as standing position. Sit comfortably in a meditative posture, where the knees can firmly touch the floor. Close your eyes and relax the body. Place the palms on the knees. Exhale completely and deeply and retain the breath outside. Perform Jalander Bandh and then contract the abdominal muscles inward and upward as much as possible. This is the Uddiyana bandha. Concentrate on the Manipur Chakra. This is the final pose. Hold as long as we are comfortable. Then slowly first release the Uddiyana bandha or abdominal contraction, then the Jalander bandha and inhale. When the respiration comes to normal, then repeat the process.

Duration: One can practice up to 10 times.

Caution: This bandha should be practiced on an empty stomach and intestines. Jalander bandha should be released before inhaling.

This bandha should not be practiced by pregnant women and person suffering from heart ailment, peptic and duodenal ulcers.

Benefits: By practicing this bandha one can get freedom from abdominal and stomach ailments like constipation, indigestion, worms, diabetes etc. The organs like liver, pancreas, kidneys, spleen are massaged and their functions improved. It stimulates the adrenal glands situated above the kidneys and Manipur chakra located in the navel region which is the center of prana in the body, hence distribution of prana is increased.

MOOL BANDHA (the perineum lock)

Sit comfortable in a meditative posture, where the knees can firmly touch the floor. Close the eyes and relax the body. Place the palms on the knees. Inhale deeply, retain the breath and perform Jalander bandha. Now contract the muscles in the perineum (or muscles of the anus) and draw them upward. Concentrate on the Mooladhar chakra. This is the final posture. Hold to this pose as long as we are comfortable holding the breath.

Then first release the perineum contraction, then the Jalander Bandh, raise the head and then slowly exhale.

Beginners may find it difficult to hold the bandh or the contractions of the perineum muscles and at the same time retain the breath. But with a little patience and practice this will be possible.

Duration: Practice 10 times or till we are comfortable holding the breath.

Benefits: The contraction of the perineum muscles facilitates the function of the intestinal peristalsis which is helpful in removal of constipation and piles. This Bandha forces the Apana Vayu in the abdominal area to flow upwards and unite with the Prana vayu in the upper chest area. This generates vitality to the entire body and helps the awakening of the Kundalini.

We have just seen how Bandha's are helpful in maintaining our physical and mental health. Now let us explore different types of 'Hasta Mudras' which are practiced while performing Asanas and Pranayama, and are also a part of Sai Ashtang Yoga.

HASTA MUDRAS:

Hasta Mudra science is a very ancient science discovered by our Rishis. According to them, the secret of health lies in the hands and fingers.

The human body is made up of 5 basic elements – earth, water, fire, air and space. When there is imbalance in these 5 elements; the body mechanism is disturbed and there is an imbalance in the body, which is the root cause of disease. The secret of good health lies in balancing these elements.

Our human body is one of the best creations of God and hands are one of the important organs of this body. A particular kind of energy in form of electromagnetic waves or electricity of the body (Aura) is continuously emitted from our hands. Hands are considered as the Health department of the body.

Hasta mudra science is a combination of fingers either touched or pressed by the thumb. By folding our fingers in a particular way or touching of hands to each other, we can cure any disturbance in the 5 elements with the help of fingers, we can keep them in proper proportion and any disturbance, excess or scarcity be balanced. By doing so our body becomes healthy.

There are many mudras performed during dance and religious functions. Here we will learn only those mudras that are helpful in curing the disorders of the body and the mind.

RELATIONSHIP BETWEEN THE 5 FINGERS AND 5 ELEMENTS:

THUMB represents FIRE
INDEX finger – AIR
MIDDLE finger – SKY
RING finger – EARTH
SMALL finger - WATER

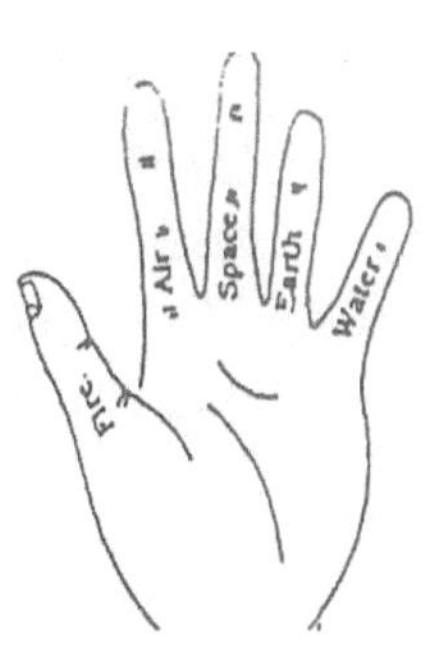

Gyan Mudra:

Touch the tip of the thumb to the tip of the index finger. Remaining fingers should be straight.

Time: This Mudra can be practiced daily.

Benefits: Helps to increase brain power, cures mental tension up to a point, anger, depression, mental concentration especially for students, sharpens memory and intelligence, certain mentally retarded children have found change in metal power. Malfunctioning of the pituitary gland can also be corrected. Regular practice of this mudra helps to develop

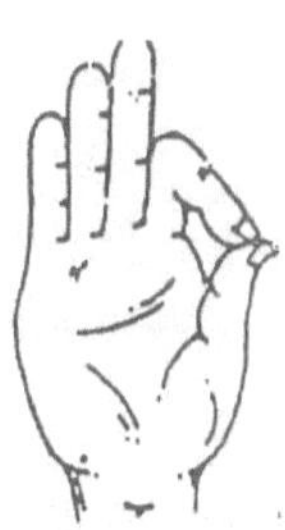

the 'sixth sense' and at times helps insomnia without the intake of sleeping tablets. Combining this mudra with Prana Mudra gives double benefit for sleeplessness and headache.

VAYU MUDRA:

Keep the Index finger at the base of the thumb, lock it with the thumb and keep the other 3 fingers straight.

Time: For regular practice 15 to 45 minutes and in acute cases 45 minutes in 12 to 24 hours.

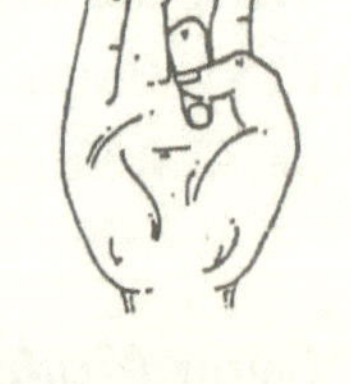

Benefits: Any pain in abdomen, neck and knee is taken care of, if this mudra is practiced regularly for a month. Cures rheumatism, gout and arthritis. Patients suffering from Parkinson's and paralysis get the much- needed boost in recovery along with other natural treatments. Blood circulation improves, all problems related to gas and windiness is taken care of.

SHUNYA MUDRA:

The middle finger is kept at the top of the mount of Venus and is pressed down with the thumb, i.e. place the middle finger at the base of the thumb and press it with the thumb.

Time: This mudra can be practiced daily for 30 to 40 minutes till improvement commences. At times relief is very rapid. However, for better result practice this mudra for 45 minutes a day with both the hands.

Benefits: Since the middle finger represents the 'space' element in the body, an increase or decrease in this element is taken care of and is balanced. It is very helpful to vertigo. When we start feeling the giddiness, we should immediately practice this mudra. Within a few minutes the problem subsides even if the problem may be chronic. All problems connected with the ears i.e. deafness, earaches, etc. are taken care of.

PRITHVI MUDRA:

The tip of the ring finger touches the tip of the thumb. The remaining fingers will be straight and relaxed.

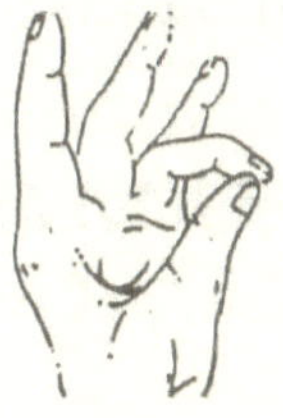

Time: This mudra can be practiced in any asana for any length of time.

Benefits:

1) It rejuvenates body and mind and increases vitality by eliminating physical weakness.
2) It gives peace of mind.
3) It increases luster of the skin and makes it glow.
4) It helps weak person to gain weight in proportion of his requirement.
5) It facilitates spiritual progress.

VARUNA MUDRA:

The tip of the little finger touches the tip of the thumb and the rest 3 fingers are straight and relaxed.

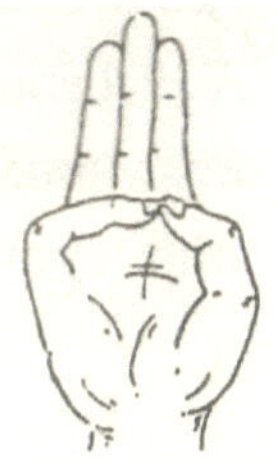

Time: As and when need, this mudra can be practiced. **Benefits:** Removes deficiency of water element, blood impurities and gastric problems and relieves pain due to cramps.

SURYA MUDRA:

Bend the ring finger and press the tip on the base of the thumb, slightly press with the thumb.

Time: Regular 5 to 15 minutes both morning and evening.

Benefits:

1) **Special benefit:** When this mudra is practiced while sitting in Padmasana, helps to reduce fats.
2) Increases heat in the body.
3) Improves digestion.

4) The pressure given on the point of the thyroid glands helps to reduce weight.

5) Relieves mental tension.

PRANA MUDRA:

The tip of the little finger and the tip of the ring finger should touch the tip of the thumb. Remaining two fingers should be straight and at ease.

Time: Practice 5 to 10 minutes with both the hands daily.

Benefits:

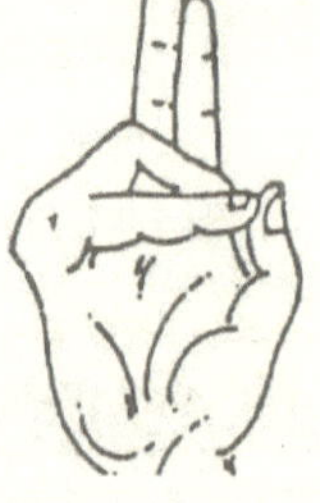

1) Keeps the eyes in a healthy state and vision improves.

2) As earth, water and fire elements are combined, there is overall increase in life force and immunity and the whole physical body is activated.

3) Brings firmness to muscles.

4) Nervousness and fatigue is eliminated.

5) Removes blockages and improves blood circulation.

6) A diabetic person with benefit by the combination of Apan mudra and Prana mudra and in Insomnia practice Prana mudra with Gyan mudra.

LINGA MUDRA:

Entangle all the fingers and keep either of the thumb erect. This mudra should be practiced in winter.

Time: As and when required.

Benefits:

1) Strengthens lungs, Relieves cold and cough both acute and chronic especially due to seasonal changes. Gives relief in bronchial attacks and good for all respiratory problems.

2) Weight reduction to a certain extent is noticed.

3) Increases heat in the body.

4) Increases resistance power in the body.

APANA MUDRA:

The tip of the middle finger and ringer finger touches the tip of the thumb while keeping the index and little finger straight.

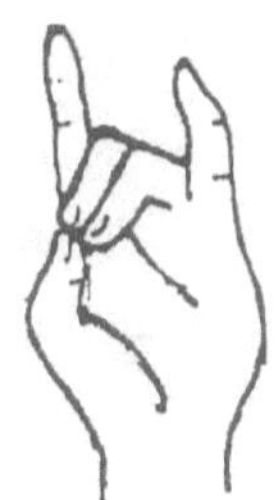

Time: As long as we want to practice and for constipation and piles 45 minutes or more regularly.

Benefits:

1) Plays an important role in regulating excretory system and keeps the body clean. It helps to clear urine and sweat regularly.
2) It reduces gas problems and cures constipation, piles and stomach aches.
3) It works as a supplementary cure in disease of the mouth, nose and eyes.
4) Apan mudra with Prithvi mudra practiced together helps the eyes.
5) Regulates the function of kidneys and also helps to control diabetes.

APANA VAYU MUDRA:

Index finger touches the base of the thumb, and the tip of the middle finger and ring finger touches the tip of the thumb. The little finger remains straight.

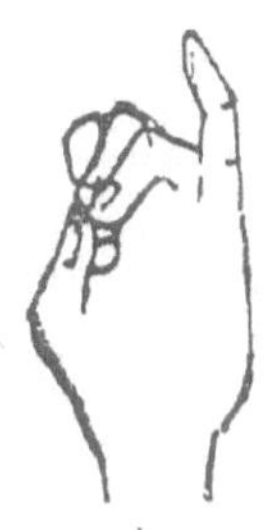

Time: Heart patients, blood pressure patients and one who has already suffered from an heart attack should practice 15 minutes morning and evening for better results and also fast recovery from surgery.

Benefits:

1) Strengthens the heart, whenever one experiences slight pain in the chest, accompanied by restlessness and pressure in the chest area, this mudra will show its effect even before the arrival of medical aid. (acts as Sorbitate to heart patients).
2) Relieves gastric troubles and regular bowl movements.

Guideline for the Practice of Mudras:

1) Mudras are easy to practice once we start practicing.

2) They are time saving as we can practice them any time, any where even while reading and writing (only with one hand), traveling, walking, watching T.V. etc.

3) If the mudra is performed by the right hand, only the left side of the body benefits and vice- versa. (Detailed explanation in Chapter Pranayama)

4) The pressure on fingers should be light. Avoid tight pressure as it will make our hands and nerves stiff.

5) At time, beginners who suffer from a particular ailment may not be able to perform a mudra with ease and flexibility. In such case one should not worry and take the help of the other hand and keep the finger in position. Gradually as one's physical problem reduces one can practice with both hands.

6) Shunya mudra and Vayu mudra should be discontinued once the problem is eradicated.

7) The time limit for any mudra is minimum 5 minutes and maximum 24 minutes which is supposed to be the best time. We can go up to 45 minutes as time permits during the day.

8) Mudras give best results when practiced along with Pranayama: inhale, retain, exhale and pause.

The 21st century with all its health problems and tribulations calls for the return to the age-old wholistic method without the use of harmful drugs as far as possible, certainly a return back to Nature.

The Asanas, Bandhas and Hasta Mudras constitute a complete set of Yogic exercises which takes care of our physical and mental health. Let us now move to the next Chapter which is a subtler aspect of Sai Ashtang Yoga namely, Pranayama.

SAI RAM

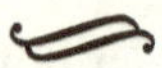

Chapter IV

Pranayama – (Breathing Techniques / Life force control)

MEANING OF PRANAYAMA

Prana means life-force and Yama means control. Pranayam means control of life-force.

Prana is our very life, the ultimate force that causes us to move, think and create, whereas breathing is only an external manifestation of Prana.

Pranayam is an exact science, it means regulation of breath or control of Prana.

It is the sum total of all the forces in nature, latent forces in us and all around us. Heat, light, electricity and magnetism are all manifestation of Prana.

By practicing Pranayama regularly, we gain the ability to direct, regulate and control the life force within us. This is done through our thinking process: thoughts are the agents who help to direct the Prana or life-force. Prana can be stored in various organs and in the chakras or energy centers and can be transferred to various organs to improve vitality, overcome disease and bring peace, serenity and enlightenment.

Yoga believes that health of the physical body not only depends on the nutritive factors but also by its content of oxygen or Prana. Pranayam super-oxidizes the blood and fully charges it with Prana. An average man breathes 15 to 18 times per minute. In normal breath cycle, you exchange 1 pint of air. By practicing Pranayam we learn to breathe deeply and automatically breathe three pints of air. Pranayam teaches us to exhale more forcefully. This allows a great supply of oxygen and Prana to be absorbed into our system.

Although medical science looks upon the body as a single vehicle with many physiological organs including a brain, Yoga looks upon the body as having three distinct vehicles, as well as consciousness.

As Sri Satya Sai rightly says – you are not one but three – the one you think you are i.e. the Physical body. What others think you are – the Mental or Astral body and what you really are – The causal body in which the Atma resides.

Prana or Pranayama is best understood in the context of sheaths. We are not one but three: the physical body, the mental body and the causal body. So Our Body, which is the temple of God (Atma) is composed of 5 sheaths and 3 bodies

<table>
<tr><td align="center">The Three Bodies</td><td align="center">The five sheaths</td></tr>
<tr><td>1)   The Physical body or Stul Sharira</td><td align="center">Annamaya Kosha – food sheath</td></tr>
<tr><td></td><td align="center">↑</td></tr>
<tr><td align="center">Connects →</td><td align="center">Pranamaya Kosha –Prana sheath</td></tr>
<tr><td></td><td align="center">↓</td></tr>
<tr><td>2)   The Mental or Astral Body or</td><td align="center">Manomaya Kosha –Mind sheath
Sukshma Sharira</td></tr>
<tr><td></td><td align="center">↑</td></tr>
<tr><td align="center">Connects →</td><td align="center">Vijnanamaya Kosha –Intellect sheath</td></tr>
<tr><td></td><td align="center">↓</td></tr>
<tr><td>3)   Causal Body or Karana Sharira</td><td align="center">Ananadmaya Kosha – Bliss sheath</td></tr>
</table>

These five sheaths and three bodies are modes and means for the expression of consciousness.

Just as there are nerves in the Physical body, there are also astral channels called Nadis in the Mental or Astral body through which the Pranic energy flows. Many people are unaware that there are life or air currents in the earth, ocean and even the sky, flowing in regulated patterns which can be charted. Just as people are unaware of the earth currents, they are also unaware of the astral currents. These life currents run throughout our physical body, in our muscular skeletal structure, the blood and the lymph system, the spinal fluids and also through the more subtle organ of the brain, known as mind.

These channels get clogged with phlegm, because of our wrong life style and wrong and negative thinking. Pranayama helps to clean and clear the channels or nadis and remove the gross and subtle phlegm. This accelerates the free flow of Prana thereby increasing physical strength, concentration and meditation. Prana also stimulates and vitalizes the gross, subtle and super-subtle levels of our being which is helpful to achieve the goal of enlightenment.

Nerve energy is one of the most important energies required for bodily and mental functions. In our day to day activities of wakefulness and dreaming this energy is continuously being used. During sleep and meditation we generate this nerve energy but during sleep, we function at a subconscious level and therefore there is no conscious control of the life energy. So how is Prana to be controlled? Prana can be controlled by practicing various breathing techniques.

The Pranic energy plays a very important role in the functions of the Manomaya Kosha or the Mental body or the sukshma sharira. The energy Centers or Chakras form a part of the Mental body namely:

1) The Mooladhar at the base of the spine, just above the anus.
2) The Swadhistan is located at the small of the back, just above the organs of procreation.
3) The Manipur lies in the navel region.
4) The Anahat lies within the Heart region.
5) The Vishuddha is located in the throat region.
6) The moon chakra is at the back of the head at the medulla oblongata.
7) The Ajna is located between the two eyebrows and is also known as the 3rd eye.
8) The Sahasrara or thousand petalled lotus is located at the top of the cerebral cavity.

The moon center at the Medulla oblongata is the door way for the Prana or the universal life-energy to enter the human body. It descends down through the cerebral spinal axis, reaches the bottom and then ascends again. This ascending and descending result in its modification by the nature of the chakras and thus the Life energy is divided into what is known as vital airs or Vayus or Panch Pranas (meaning 5 Pranas).

As the soul or Atma passes innumerable of times through the cycle of birth and death; there is a collection of desires, by the Ego or false self. They are desires to survive or live, to enjoy, to create etc. which forms into a strong knot at the Mooladhar or root Chakra and is called the Brahma Ghat or Granthi. All the attachments that the Ego or false self, gathers, such as the feeling of 'me' and 'mine' gets collected and is set in form of a knot at the Anahat or Heart Chakra and is known as Vishnu Ghat or Granthi. The spell of illusion or Maya or Ego creates the knot of ignorance at the Ajna chakra or the 3rd eye and is known as the Shiv Ghat or Granthi. With the help of Pranayama and other breathing techniques these knots are loosed, which is a great step in our spiritual progress.

FUNCTIONS OF BREATH OR PRANA
There are 72,000 Nerve centers/nadies in our body.

a) The air/oxygen that we inhale flows through these Nerve centers and controls our nervous system (Physical Body)

b) The air/Prana that we inhale flows through the Nadis (subtle form of Nerves) and controls the energy centers or Chakras. (Mental Body).

3 Main Nadies

PINGLA –SURYA NADI:-	Right Nostril, Positive side of the body or Yang – connected with Physical Actions
IDA – CHANDRA NADI:-	Left Nostril, Negative side of the body or Yin – connected with Mental Activities.
CENTRE MARIDIAN: - **OR**	Connects all the chakras from Muladhar to Sahasrara. Connected with Spiritual activities.
SUSHMNA NADI	**Balances both Surya and Chandra Nadies.**

During His Divine Discourse at Sai Kulvant Hall on Vinayak Chatruthi day on 25/8/2009 Swami spoke thus:

"It is a fact that people cannot live without air. It is the very life principle of not only humans, but of all living beings. Lord Vinayaka permeates this life principle. He is the very embodiment of our breath. He is the SOHAM TATTWA, verily. The breathing process consists of three actions – Puraka (inhaling), Kumbhaka (holding the breath) and Rechaka (exhaling). The regulation of these three actions is called Pranayama. The processes of inhaling, retention and exhaling of the air must be regulated in such a way that equal time is taken for each process and the entire exercise is done in a natural manner without any strain. Then only DHYANA (meditation) is possible. Lord Vinayaka is the presiding deity of Pranayama. He confers Vidya (education) and Siddhi (success in aim) on people. That is why he is extolled as SIDDHI VINAYAKA. These two are of utmost importance to human being. Since, there is none to explain this secret; people celebrate the festival of Vinayaka Chaturthi in a casual manner without realizing its underlying significance.

Diagram showing the Panch Pranas in our body.

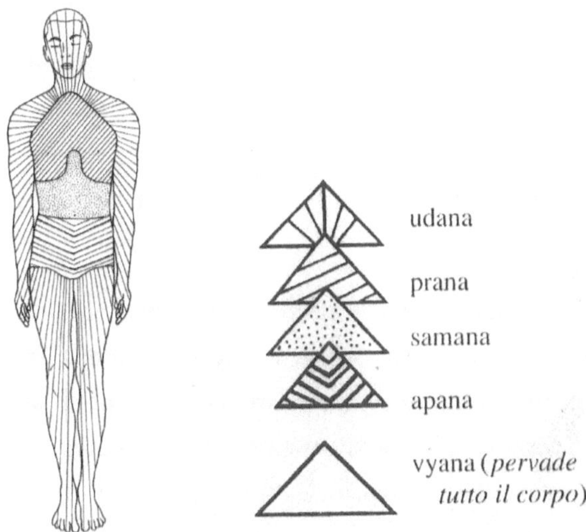

PANCH PRANA:

Traditionally, the prana in the body is divided into five elementary parts which are collectively known as Panch Prana. They consist of Prana, Apana, Samana, Udana and Vyana.

- **PRANA:** This Prana Vayu is located between the larynx and the diaphragm. It is the vital energy by which breathe is drawn inside. It is connected with the functions of the heart, lungs, speech and throat. It helps to carry the food and drink to the stomach. One should not confuse the Life Energy Prana with this modified prana (which is a part of the Panch Prana). This Prana manifest itself as So-Hum and its activities are centered in the Anahat or Heart Chakra.

- **APANA:** This is located below the navel region up to the anus and provides energy to the large intestine, kidneys, anus and genitals. This vital force carries out waste products like urine and stools and is concerned with the expulsion of prana through rectum and the nose and the mouth. The apana has a downward flow. This energy relates to and circulates through the Mooladhar or root chakra.

- **SAMANA:** This is located within the region in between the Heart and navel. It is associated with the Manipur Chakra and regulates the functions of digestive system, liver, intestines, pancreas, stomach, heart, circulatory system and the secretions they supply. It helps in the assimilation of food.

- **VYANA:** This vital force pervades the entire body and controls the upward and downward flow of the Prana and Apana but which centers in the Swadhistan chakra. It regulates and controls all the movements of the body and harmonizes and activates the limbs and their associated muscles, ligaments, nerves and joints. It is also responsible for the metabolic rate and the erect posture of the body.

- **UDANA:** This force is located above the larynx and manifests through the Vishuddhi Chakra. It regulates the functions of the eyes, nose, ears and all sensory receptors. It regulates the diaphragm and thus the depth and rhythm of respiration. Udana is very important especially at the time of death; its function is to release the astral body from the hold of the physical body. This can be better understood by the manifestation of the death rattle, a peculiar sound in the throat sometimes heard at the time of a person's death. Without Udana we would be unable to be conscious of the outside world.

PANCH UPAPRANAS:

There are also five Upapranas, namely Naga, Koorma, Krikara, Devadatta and Dhananjaya.

The Naga is associated with belching and alertness; the koorma is responsible for the action of blinking; the Krikara is related with sneezing, scratching, hunger and thirst; the Devadatta is associated with hiccupping and depression and Dhananjaya is connected with yawning and sounds generated due to the passage of wind from the anus and movements of the joints. Dhananjaya is the last of the upaprana which leaves the body resulting in bloating after death.

The Flow Pattern of the Energy Level in Our Body

Just as the ocean has high tides and low tides, similarly Prana flows in and out of our Physical and Astral bodies. At sunrise, prana enters the Center channel or Sushumna Nadi; at noon it flows equally both in the Physical and Astral body; at sunset it rushes through the physical arteries or blood stream and at midnight it rests in the blood vessels and the hollow of the heart.

The circulation of Prana in the blood and the physical energies are at a peak from 12 noon to 12 midnight. From midnight until noon it is polarized in the Nadis. Intellectual activity is much sharper and at its peak at this time. Therefore, post midnight and wee early morning hours are preferred by creative artist in all ages, all countries and all faculties for their creative work.

Guidelines for Pranayama

1) The practice of Pranayama must be undertaken in a clean, well ventilated and pleasant environment.

2) Sit on a blanket or a cushion on the floor, for the practice. One can use a flat chair with a thin cushion on it.

3) Pranayama should be practiced on an empty stomach or after 4 hours of breakfast or meals.

4) Our body should be completely relaxed and the spine, neck and head should be erect and centered. Siddhasana, Padmasana, Siddha Yoni asana are the best poses for Pranayama but if one is finding it difficult then one may even practice in Ardha Padmasana.

5) During the practice of Pranayama, one should not strain. The breath should not be retained for longer than is comfortable. This is important as our lungs are very delicate and misuse can cause them injury. Take precaution not to bloat the abdomen during inhalation because this is the key factor in all Pranayamas.

6) Sit facing East or north for the practice of Pranayama which is helpful for polar effect. Pranayam should be practiced with regularity; in the same posture, same place and at approximately the same time each day.

7) Pranayam can be practiced at any time but the ancient texts point out that pranayama should be practiced 4 times a day. This is difficult for a working person so it is suggested that 15 minutes in the morning and 15 minutes in the evening will produce excellent benefits and also spiritual unfoldment.

8) If we come across any difficulty or problem, consult an expert Yoga teacher.

9) Pranayama should be avoided if one is suffering from fever, headache, constipation or loose bowels. In the beginning there are chances we may feel constipated and there could be a reduction in the quantity of urine. Drink a good amount of water and reduce salt and spices in your diet.

10) Those practicing intense Pranayama should not use tobacco or drink alcohol.

11) If we perspire during the practice of Pranayama, rub the sweat into the skin with our palms or let it dry of its own. Do not use a fan or wipe it off with our clothes.

12) Beginners should not practice heat producing Pranayamas during summer and cold producing Pranayamas during winter.

13) Complete fasting or single meal is not advisable for Pranayama practitioners. Always have some milk, butter or ghee with lunch or dinner and avoid hard, dry, stale or spicy food items.

14) For higher type of Pranayama, always seek the direct guidance of a master.

15) During the practice of pranayama there should be no tension either caused by Yogic posture or by any mental apprehensions. An accumulation of saliva in the mouth usually indicates a state of tension. If there is accumulation we need to relax the body and the mind before beginning pranayama, Another important point is do not swallow the saliva while holding the breath, we cannot swallow and continue to hold the breath. So swallow the saliva immediately after exhalation.

16) If pressure is felt in the ears or heavy ringing is heard, either slowdown or stop the pranayama for a while.

17) Practice of pranayama is best done sitting on the floor as it lowers our blood pressure etc. However if not possible a chair is acceptable. The eyes should remain closed during the entire process for two reasons. Firstly, keeping eyes open may result in burning sensation and secondly, our mind will wander scattering the pranic energies and we will not be able to concentrate.

18) Whenever there is exhaustion, do not practice Pranayama.

Benefits of Pranayama

1) Pranayam helps to take Prana to various parts of the body, better and helps to restore the body to good health and also restores the mind to a peaceful state.

2) It helps for concentration and contemplation and also gives us a certain amount of inner vision (intuition). Thus is helpful in meditation.

3) With the help of Pranayama we can control breathing, which regulates the subtle Prana. With the control of Prana, mind can be controlled. Thus,

BREATH → CONTROLS → PRANA → CONTROLS → MIND

The vibration of the Prana produces THOUGHTS in the mind. Prana moves the mind. Ex. Gold smith removes the impurities of gold by heating the gold in hot furnace by blowing the blow pipe; similarly by Pranayama we can remove the impurities of the body and indriyas or senses.

Like metals purified over fire in the crucible, the slag of karma is removed by Pranayama and the mind is freed from contamination. The MIND AND BODY are both rendered PURE.

4) The body's resistance power improves and Pranayama helps to eliminate all diseases and adjust easily to different climates and therefore we can achieve perfect health.

5) With the help of Pranayama and Kumbhaka (retention of breath), the body reaches a state of stability which is very helpful for higher stages of meditation and Samadhi.

6) We can achieve special powers like levitation, moving in space and can reach a stage of no- mind with the mastery of Pranayama.

7) With regular practice of Pranayama and Kumbhaka, we can live longer than the average age. The average number of breaths for the average human being is twelve to fifteen per minute. If we reduce the number of breaths per minutes, we extends the life span. When the breath is retained or suspended (Kumbhaka) it increases the inner spiritual vigor.

8) Scientific research claims that only 3% of the grey matter within the nervous system of the brain is utilized by an average person. This means a very small percentage of the massive gray matter within your body is stimulated and used in our day-to-day life. With the practice of Pranayama, the inhaled oxygen is absorbed more rapidly on the surface of the muscles than on the nerves, producing a static electrical charge. While

practicing Pranayama techniques, we focus heavily at the cerebral regions which drives more blood in that direction.

The static electricity follows the normal flow of blood, which acts as a catalyst or stimulus in awakening a greater quantity of brain cells or the gray matter. With the activation of more brain cells comes greater perception, greater retention, greater recalling capacity, greater creativity, greater positivity and happiness.

9) Pranayama helps to remove the phlegm and impurities and charges the blood stream with oxygen which revitalizes the nerves when practiced regularly. This helps the dormant brain cells to reopen producing an expansion of consciousness known as Cosmic Consciousness.

10) By the practice of pranayama there is a marked change in mental attitude and mental outlook, which includes reduction of fears, a reduction in cravings, increase in creative imagination, optimistic outlook and a great ability to concentrate.

Impact of Pranayam on Longevity:

a) Pranayama promotes slow and rhythmic breathing and the objective of promoting slow and rhythmic breathing is that it is said that the longevity of life is said to increase when we slow our breathing process.

b) An average person, without any knowledge of breath control, will probably take 15 breaths per minute i.e. 21,600 breaths per day (10800 inhalations and 10800 exhalations)

c) A Yogi or a spiritual aspirant will take around 6 to 7 breaths per minute.

d) Longer the breath, deeper and less number of breaths, the life span is more. Shorter the breath and more number of breaths, the life span is shorter.

Ex. A tortoise lives more than 200 years and a dog or a rabbit lives shorter life.

It is estimated that a monkey is short lived because it takes 40 breaths per minute, whereas a snake lives longer because it takes around 3 to 4 breaths per minutes. Hence, one of the objectives of breath management is to reduce the number of breaths/minute that we take.

Perfect Breathing

Most of the time we use only half of our lung capacity to breathe because of our shallow breathing. Because of this our body and brain are deprived of proper amount of oxygen. We cannot live without breathing, but by half breathing we only half live.

Secondly, most of us breathe incorrectly. When we inhale our abdomen contracts and when we exhale our abdomen expands. This is a totally incorrect way of breathing.

Abdominal Breathing: We can experience if our breathing is correct by placing our hand on the navel. Inhale deeply; our hand will rise as the abdomen expands. The diaphragm is a strong muscle which separates the lungs from the abdominal organs. The lower it moves during inhalation, the more air is inhaled into the lungs.

Exhale deeply and the hand moves down as the abdomen contracts and the diaphragm moves higher. Maximum air is expelled from the lungs. Our chest and shoulders should not move during this practice.

Chest Breathing or Thoracic Breathing: Inhale while expanding the chest, so that the ribs move outward and upward. Exhale and the ribs will move inward and downward. Try not to move the abdomen at all.

Perfect Breathing: Perfect breathing is the combination of the two breathing patterns mentioned above. With the practice of this breathing it is possible to inhale maximum air or oxygen and exhale maximum amount of air or carbon dioxide. This is the correct way to breathe:

Inhale deeply by expanding the abdomen and then the chest in one slow, smooth motion until our lungs have drawn the maximum amount of air.

Exhale by first relaxing the chest and then the abdomen. Finally accentuate the contraction of the abdominal muscles, so that the maximum amount of air is expelled from the lungs. The complete procedure of inhalation and exhalation should be very smooth.

Initially, we may have to practice this correct way of breathing consciously for a few minutes every day, preferably before starting Pranayama. Eventually, the process will become automatic and should be done throughout the day.

Because of the highly improved quality of breathing, our vitality will improve and we will be less susceptible to minor illnesses like cough and cold. Our thinking power improves and there will be less anxiety and stress.

The Basic Divisions in All Pranayama:

All the Pranayamas are basically divided into four factors known as: (1) Puraka (2) Rechaka (3) Antar Kumbhaka and (4) Bahir Kumbhaka.

1) **PURAKA: (Inhalation)** Puraka means, when we inhale air deeply, either through left nostril, right nostril, both the nostrils or sometimes through the mouth. During inhalation, fill and expand the upper abdomen and then the chest up to the neck. The Prana spreads in between this region. In simple words it is called **Inhalation.**

2) **RECHAKA: (Exhalation)** Rechak means when we very slowly exhale through the left nostril, the right nostril, both nostrils or through the mouth. In Pranayama, Rechaka is very important as it eliminates maximum toxins from the body. The lower abdomen is the seat of Apana, the area of impurities in the body and the navel is the seat of fire element. More emphasis is given to exhalation so that the Apana rises up to the navel for the burning of impurities. In unconscious breathing this is low whereas in Pranayama it is very high. Exhalation has also a calming and relaxing effect.

3) **ANTAR KUMBHAKA: (Internal Retention)** Retaining the breath inside, after inhalation for a definite period, comfortably as per the capacity of the practitioner is called Antar Kumbhaka. During this process, Prana spreads to the whole body or as directed by our own thinking.

4) **BAHIR KUMBHAKA: (External Retention)** After complete exhalation, holding the breath outside, comfortably for a definite period as per the capacity of the practitioner is called Bahir Kumbhaka.

Though the above mentioned factors seem like separate functions they are in close connection with each other. The change in one factor influences the other, for example if the inhalation is long, then the exhalation becomes short and fast and if the inner retention is longer it effects the exhalation and outer retention. Thus in different Pranayama all the above factors change and play differing roles in the removal of impurities. Therefore we should first understand and then commence with the practice of Pranayama

Practice of Pranayama

Here are two very simple but very useful Pranayamas, namely Surya Nadi Pranayama and Chandra Nadi Pranayama.

Surya Nadi Pranayama

Sit in a comfortable position, head straight, spine erect, eyes closed and body relaxed.

Close the left nostril with the thumb of the left hand. Inhale slowly and deeply through the right nostril and without holding or retention of the breath exhale slowly and deeply through the same i.e. right nostril. In short, inhale and exhale slowly and deeply only through the right nostril i.e. the Surya Nadi. Repeat this process 10 times, rest for some time and again repeat the process 10 times. We can practice more rounds when we feel comfortable.

Benefits: This Pranayama gives fast relief from cold and cough and headaches. It creates more heat in the body hence it is good when practiced during winter season. One should reduce the practice of this Pranayama in summer.

Caution: People with acidity problem should not practice this Pranayama.

Chandra Nadi Pranayama

Sit in a comfortable position, head straight, spine erect, eyes closed and body relaxed.

Close the right nostril with the thumb of the right hand. Inhale slowly and deeply through the left nostril and without holding or retention of the breath exhale slowly and deeply through the same i.e. left nostril. In short, inhale and exhale slowly and deeply only through the left nostril i.e. the Chandra Nadi. Repeat this process 10 times, rest for some time and again repeat the process 10 times. We can practice more rounds when we feel comfortable.

Benefits: This pranayama has a very cooling effect in the entire system. It cures acidity. This pranayama should be practiced more in summer than winter.

Caution: People suffering from frequent cold problems should not practice this exercise

Both the above mentioned pranayama, when practiced regularly, keeps the body's heat and cold balance maintained.

Sahaja Pranayama:

This is a very simple type of pranayama, which is very useful if practiced just before meditation. It collects our thoughts and brings our mind to one-pointedness faster. It causes the mind to be steady and clear and we gain great power of concentration.

Sit in a comfortable meditative posture and form the surrender Mudra (The tip of the index finger should touch the center of the thumb and the rest three fingers should be kept straight) with the left hand, placing it on the left knee. Place the right hand thumb on the right nostril and close the right nostril. Slowly inhale through the left nostril, mentally counting 3, hold the breath and count 12. While doing so our point of focus should be at the Ajna Chakra. Now with the ring finger and little finger close the left nostril and release the thumb from the right nostril and slowly exhale counting 6. Now repeat the same process with the right nostril. The two processes together constitute one round, and such 6 rounds constitute one cycle. After we are comfortable with this ratio of 3:12:6, we can slowly increase the ratio by one point i.e. 4:16:8 so and so forth.

One should practice this Pranayama at least 2 times (and then increase the rounds) daily before starting meditation. Just as we do Ganesh Pooja before we start any auspicious work, this pranayama symbolizes Ganesh Pooja before meditation as Ganapati is Pranavaswaroopa. i.e.Ganapati is Pranava or Prana or our life force himself. This definitely makes a very big difference during meditation.

Savitri Pranayama

This is a very different type of Pranayama but a very important one for one's spiritual progress. This practice should be done after the above-mentioned Sahaja pranayama and start with the meditation.

Sit in a comfortable meditative posture and form the surrender mudra. First finish with the Sahaja Pranayam and then start with Savitri Pranayama.

Focus our awareness or attention on our feet and as we inhale with both the nostrils, slowly lift our awareness mentally from our feet to the Ajna chakra or 3rd eye, mentally chanting Aum, but take a little pause at the Mooladhar chakra and when we reach the Ajna chakra mentally chant Bhuh.. and then exhale. We have to continue mentally chanting Om (only once) till you reach the ajan chakra. E.g. Oooooooo…….mmm Bhuh. Repeat this 5 times. Then repeat the same procedure lifting our awareness from the feet, mentally chanting Om to Ajna Chakra but this time pausing at the Swadhistan Chakra and when we reach at the Ajna Chakra mentally chant Bhuwah… and then exhale. Repeat this 5 times. Similarly continue the same process, till we reach the Ajna chakra and when we come to the last chakra i.e. Sahasrara chakra, the awareness should be carried up to the crown of the head and either end the process there or bring the awareness back to the Ajna Chakra, whichever is comfortable. Given below is an illustration showing the position of the chakras.

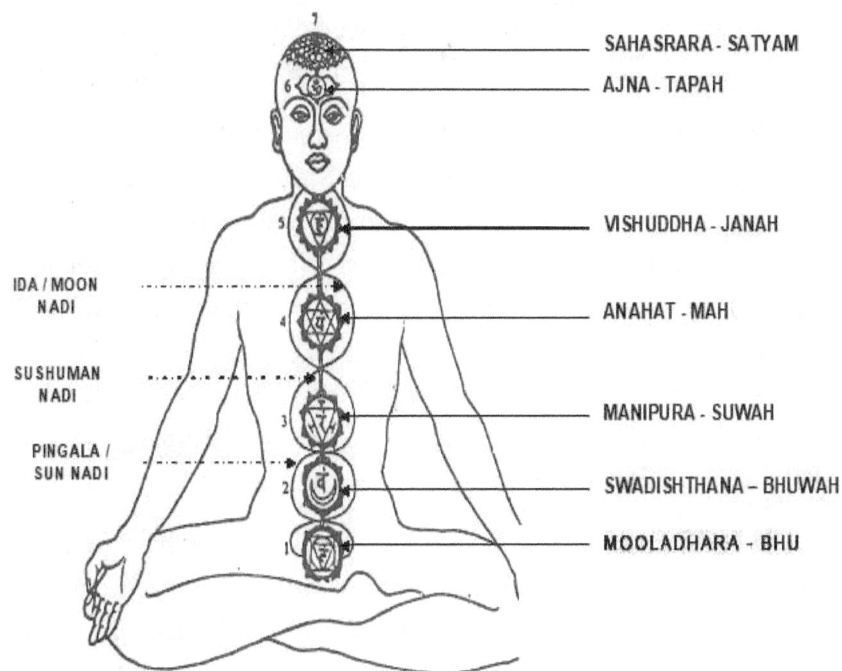

Given bellow are the names of the chakras and their respective chants.

CHAKRA	CHANTS
Mooladhara	Om Bhuwah..
Swadhistana	Om Bhuwah…
Manipura	Om Suwaha…
Anahat	Om Maha
Vishudhha	Om Janah
Ajna	Om Tapah
Sahasrara	Om Satyam

After completing the entire process, start with the meditation. There will be great focus on the Ajna chakra and our concentration will be steady and better.

Note: The main purpose of this pranayama is to lift our consciousness (which is omnipresent and is spread out in our whole body) from the feet to the

3rd eye. To lift the consciousness the vehicle used is Om or Pranava. This not only helps us in concentration but also we progress faster in meditation.

OMKAR: (also known as Udageeta Pranayama) Om, the Vedic mantra is the primal sound and rightly known as the Shabdabrahma. It is the sound of the creation. It is the mother of all mantras and is the Bij Mantra of the Ajna chakra and prefixes most mantras. Om is the symbol of wisdom for it is the vibratory sound of Brahman- The ultimate truth or reality. It is written as AUM but actually chanted as O-mmm. AUM represents the trinity, 'A' represents creator the Brahma, 'U' represents sustainer, Vishnu and 'M' represents dissolver, Mahesha. It also harmonizes the Trigunas – Satva, Rajas and Tamas by which all is balanced well.

The energy centers or the Chakras in our Astral body also have Bij Mantras. They are as follows – Mooladhar – LAM, Swadhistan – VAM, Manipur – RAM, Anahat – YAM, Vishudha – HAM, and finally the Ajan Chakra – AUM or OM.

We will observe that all these Bij mantras end in AM. So chanting of AUM energizes all the chakras or energy centers having a very positive effect on our mind and body. Secondly the main astral channels, the Ida or Chandra Nadi (left side) and Pingala or Surya Nadi (right side) and the Sushumna intersect at 7 places. Hence 3 channels or Nadis intersecting at 7 places is 7x3=21. Therefore number 21 is given importance.

Hence when AUM is chanted 21 times it gives the required positive effect on all the chakras which in turn has a very significant effect on our mind and body.

Practice of Aum

Sit in a comfortable posture. Take 2 deep breaths to relax the body and mind. Then inhale deeply and while exhaling slowly chant A….U….M till we have completely exhaled. Again inhale deeply and chant, continue doing so for 21 times.

If we chant "A" for a prolonged time it will affect our physical level. Our desires will be fulfilled; we will be respected by all. Our mind and intellect will develop which will present us as a very positive and pleasing personality. We will be energetic and succeed in all walks of life. While chanting AUM if we put more stress on "U"; that will affect our mental level. There will be an extra ordinary development in our intelligence and we will attain superior knowledge. If we chant "M" for a longer time; it will affect our spiritual level. It will purify the mind and we will have better and faster spiritual development.

Bhasrika Pranayam: (the Bellows Breath)

Sit comfortably in a meditative asana with the spine erect and head held at 90° from the ground or the head should be held straight. Close our eyes and completely relax our body. Both hands should be in Vayu Mudra (The index finger should be at the base of our thumb and the thumb should rest on the index finger. The other 3 fingers should be kept open.) and rest on both the knees respectively.

Inhale forcefully and deeply with both the nostrils and again exhale forcefully and completely without retaining the breath. Inhaling and exhaling makes 1 cycle. Repeat 10 to 12 cycles. When we are comfortable with 12 cycles, practice for 1 minute. This will be considered as one round. Rest for a short while before we commence the second round. In this technique the lungs are used liked a blacksmith's bellows and hence it is called the bellows breath. Beginners should practice this exercise slowly for the first few weeks and gradually increase the speed of respiration as the lungs become stronger.

This forceful breathing directs the Prana Energy to the brain and to our entire face and we will sense a tinkling feeling all over our face. During the rest period we may say some positive affirmations mentally, which prove to be very beneficial.

Duration: This Pranayama creates heat in the body hence should be practiced only for 3 to 5 minutes per day.

Precautions: If one experiences the feeling of faintness or perspiration; it indicates that the exercise is not performed correctly. Stop the practice till our body is fit for the same. Violent shaking of the body, facial contortions and violent respiration should be avoided. If there is throbbing in the ears or bleeding through the nose, then stop the practice immediately. Practice other Pranayamas till we strengthen our body and then resume this pranayama.

Limitations: People suffering from high or low blood pressure, heart ailments, vertigo, glaucoma, pus in the ears, should not practice this Pranayama.

Benefits: It is the best way to purify the lungs, unwanted gases and germs. It helps in curing asthma, tuberculosis inflammation of the throat; it works as an expectorant and expels the accumulated phlegm. It increases appetite and brings peace and tranquility to the mind.

Kapalabhatti Pranayam

Sit in a comfortable meditative posture, with head straight and spine erect. Eyes should be closed and body should be completely relaxed.

To start with, expel the breath completely. Inhale normally and exhale forcefully. In this technique the inhalation is spontaneous while the exhalation is forceful. Start the practice and do the Jalandhar Bandh and continue the practice with the bandh. In the beginning practice only 20 exhalations and as we begin to get comfortable gradually increase the exhalation. With continuous practice we can practice up to 200 exhalations at a time. Approximately 300 exhalations would make 5 minutes if the rate of one exhalation is one second.

Duration: 10 to 15 minutes per day.

Benefits: This Pranayama affects all the organs below the abdominal area positively. It cures asthma, indigestion, stomach ailments, ailments connected with the reproductory system and relieves one of cerebral thrombosis. It reduces fats round the abdominal area. It also affects the metabolic rate, which helps in balancing the overall weight of the body, i.e. fat people reduce weight and slim people will put on weight. This Pranayama purifies the frontal region of the brain. It revitalizes the mind and keeps it cool and calm. It also balances tridoshas – Vat, Pitha and Khof.

Tri-bandha or Bhayya Pranayama

This Pranayama should be practiced immediately after the Kapalabhati Pranayama because the energy gets collected at the Mooladhara after the practice of Kapalabhati. When Tri-bandha is practiced, a vacuum is created; the energy rushes upward and is distributed in the entire body.

Sit in the same position as Kapalabhati. First completely exhale the air through both the nostrils, and immediately perform the tri-bandha; Moola bandha or anal contraction, Uddiyan bandha or stomach contraction and Jalander Bandha or chin lock contraction.

Hold this 3 positions as long as we are comfortable or we may count till 10 and then release the 3 bandhas, first the Jalander bandha, then the Udddiyan bandha and lastly the Mool bandha one after the other and slowly inhale. This is one round. Perform 3 rounds.

Benefits: Equal distribution of energy throughout the body. It increases concentration and steadies the mind.

Aulomvilom Pranayama

Sit in a comfortable meditative posture with spine erect and head held high. Eyes should be closed and body completely relaxed.

Close the right nostril with the right hand thumb, and inhale through the left nostril normally. Then immediately close the left nostril with the ring and little finger, release the thumb on the right nostril and exhale from the right nostril. Again inhale from the right nostril, close the right nostril and release the two fingers on the left nostril and exhale through the left nostril. There is no holding or retention of the breath. The inhalation and exhalation should be equal. This makes one round. Always begin with the left nostril. Care should be taken to see that we do not bloat the stomach after we inhale. The inhalation should fill the chest area and not the stomach area.

Continue the process for 1 minute, stop for some time and when our breathing becomes normal then continue the practice.

Duration: The duration should be same as Kapalabhati Pranayama. If Kapalabhati is practiced for 10 minutes then Anulomvilom should also be practiced for 10 minutes.

Benefits: This pranayams cures the illnesses of the chest area, like asthma, cold and cough, Upper respiratory tract infections, heart ailment, high and low blood pressures, nerve disorders. It increases the power of concentration and retention, keeps the brain and mind alert i.e. it increases our awareness. This Pranayama balances the Vat, Pitha and Khof or the tridosha in our body.

Note: Bhasrika, Kapalabhati and Anulomvilom are very important Pranayama. Bhasrika provides oxygen and Prana to the brain and mind respectively, Kapalabhati takes care of the lower part of the abdomen and Anulomvilom takes care of the upper part of the body. Hence they should be practiced in the same order as given above daily for good physical and mental health.

Bhramari Pranayam

Sit in a comfortable meditative posture, head straight and spine erect. Eyes should be closed and body completely relaxed.

Plug both the ears with the thumb of both the hands, the index finger of both the hands should be on the forehead, above the beginning of the eyebrows, the middle fingers should be just below the eyebrows near the stem of the nose and the ring and the little fingers should be used to close both the eyelids. This forms the complete posture for Bhramari Pranayam. Now inhale deeply with both the nostrils and as we exhale hum the word AUM or OM slowly till we completely exhale. This is one round. Again inhale...... Repeat the process. The exhalation should be slow and steady. Feel the sound vibrations in the brain and be conscious only of the sound.

Duration: Start with 5 rounds and slowly increase the number of rounds.

Benefits: Eliminates throat ailments, cures insomnia, improves the voice quality, relieves mental tension and anxiety, reduces the blood pressure, it quiets the mind and increases concentration. With regular practice we can hear the Om sound at Psychic level and helps you in meditation.

Udageeta Pranayama

Udageeta Pranayama and omkar is the same. (Please refer to Omkar).

Ujjayi Pranayama

Sit in a comfortable position, head straight and spine erect, eyes closed and body relaxed.

Contract the glottis in the throat; fold the tongue back so that the underside of the tongue is pressed against the back of the upper palate. Inhale slowly and deeply though both the nostrils making a 's-s-a- a-a' sound as the air passes through the contracted glottis. Do not bloat the stomach. Fill the air only in the upper portion of the lungs and then perform Jalander Bandh. Hold as long as one is comfortable and then close the right nostril with the right thumb and slowly exhale through the left nostril. The exhalation should also be felt in the throat (exhalation can be done by either nostrils). This constitutes one round.

Duration: Can be practiced from 3 minutes to 9 minutes.

Benefits: It has soothing effect on the entire nervous system, calms the mind, it is very helpful for people suffering from Thyroid problems, insomnia, high blood pressure and any other pulmonary diseases. Aging process is slowed down.

Sheetali Pranayama

Sit in any comfortable meditative posture, body relaxed and palms on the knees. Extend the tongue and fold the sides to form a narrow tube. Inhale slowly and deeply through the folded tongue till the abdomen and chest is completely filled with air. Retain the breath for short time and perform Jalander bandh. After a short time, release the Jalander bandh and exhale through the nose.

The formation of the tube-shape of the tongue, cools the air as it is inhaled, which has a cooling effect on the whole body system. This pranayama should be avoided in very cold winters.

Duration: Start with 5 rounds and can extend upto 50 rounds.

Benefits: Cools the entire system. Quenches thirst, purifies blood, and gives mental tranquility.

Sheetkari Pranayama

This Pranayama is similar to the above sheetali pranayama, except the position of the tongue. In Sheetkari pranayama the tongue should be folded back so that the tip of the lower surface of the tongue touches the upper palate. Clench the teeth and spreading the lips as much as possible, inhale through the mouth, till the abdomen and chest is completely filled with air. Retain the breath for a short while and perform the Jalander Bandha. After a short while release the Jalander bandh and exhale through the nose.

This Pranayama also give the entire system, the cooling effect, and should be avoided in very cold winters.

Duration and Benefits are same as above.

So far we have discussed, the four outer Angas or limbs or steps of the Sai Ashtang Yoga. Now let us explore the next four inner steps, starting with Pratyahar or sense control or sense withdrawal in our next Chapter.

SAI RAM

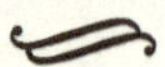

Chapter V
Pratyahar – (Sense Withdrawal)

Having studied and practiced the Outer steps of Yoga: Yama, Niyam, Asana and Pranayama. We now move to the inner steps, i.e. Pratyahara – Sense Withdrawal, Dharana – Concentration, Dhyana – Meditation and Samadhi.

HOW OUR PSYCHOLOGY FUNCTIONS:

Our total awareness, which is also known as **CHITTA,** constitutes the **MIND STUFF,** i.e. the mind which is conscious, unconscious, subconscious, preconscious and super conscious.

This Chitta is composed of 3 separate functions, which as per the scriptures is called the

Antakaran.
1) Mind or Sense Organs (Manas)
2) Intellect (Buddhi)
3) Ego (Ahamkar)

The brain → gross organs linked → external sense organs i.e. Karmendriyas are the ears, skin, eyes, tongue and nose convey the external experience of the external objects to the mind and intellect.

The subtle organs- Jyanendriyas also experience these objects and convey this experience to the mind, which is transferred to the intellect where these experiences are converted into data and knowledge. Then it is evaluated by the Ego and if found acceptable, is bought up into Consciousness.

The subtle organs are called Chakras and classify everything into 10 categories.

1) Muladhara	Shani Chakra	Duty and continent, root Earthing i.e. gravitational Pull.
2) Swadhistana	Guru Chakra	Expansion, creation
3) Manipur	Mangal Chakra	Energy and Lower Emotion
4) Anahat	Shukra Chakra	Classifies love feelings an Emotion.
5) Vishudha	Budh Chakra	Ego, creativity, oratory
6) Ajna	Ravi Chakra	Music, artists etc. Thinking, thought processes, 3rd eye etc.
7) Medulla oblongata Sahasrara	Moon or Chandra Chakra Thousand Petal Lotus	Entry point of Prana

THE PATHWAY OF PRANA

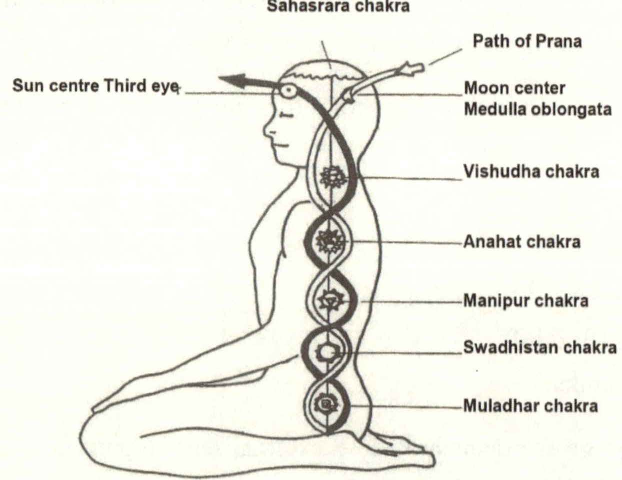

Each Chakra has a Solar and Lunar side

As we inhale, the Prana comes in at the moon centre descends through the 5 lower chakras and then ascends back through the 5 lower chakras, but on the other side. It then radiates out through the Sun Center.

The sun and moon chakras do not play a part in modifying this life energy. They are referred as luminaries or solar and lunar forces. As Prana ascends and descends through the solar and lunar sides, each of the chakras does become modified. At this time, energy is mystically modified or charged just as magnetism produces electricity, electricity produces light or light produces heat, this modified energy is known as Vital force or Shakti.

These chakras, when created, were divided into two segments:

a) An incoming feminine state and

b) Outgoing masculine state. Hence,

7. **THE THOUSAND PETTALLED LOTUS**
    Transcends the six lower realms

6. **AJNA Chakra**   - The feminine side of your Consciousness is **Cancer**
                          - The masculine side of your Consciousness is **Leo**

5. **VISHUDHA**   - The masculine side is **Gemini**
                          - The feminine side is **Virgo**

4. **ANAHAT**   - The feminine side is **Taurus**
                          - The masculine side is **Libra**

3. **MANIPUR**   - The masculine side is **Aries**
                          - The feminine side is **Scorpio**

2. **SWADISHSTAN**   - The feminine side is **Pisces**
                          - The masculine side is **Sagittarius**

1. **MULADHAR**   - The masculine side is **Aquarius**
                          - The feminine side is **Capricorn**

These above 5 chakras are male and female. Thus there are 10 storage areas; each is sensitive to one of the ten Pranic Energies (Pancha Prana and Panch Upaprana).

On the deeper level the 10 Pranic energies move through the 5 lower chakras and activate them.

All the Yoga, all mysticism, ultimately comes back to the utilization and control of these forces. It involves balancing of Prana and those 10 chakras.

Though these seem to look like separate processes, they are actually only one, comprising the totality of **MIND STUFF (CHITTA)**

Mind Stuff or Chitta is the totality of Consciousness, which includes the mind or sense organs, intelligence and the Ego. The Chitta functions through the trigunas, namely Tamas- lethargy, Rajas or Passionate activity and Sattva or Compassionate activity, respectively. All the three function as one process and this is known as the **ANTAKARAN.**

The Function of the Antakaran:

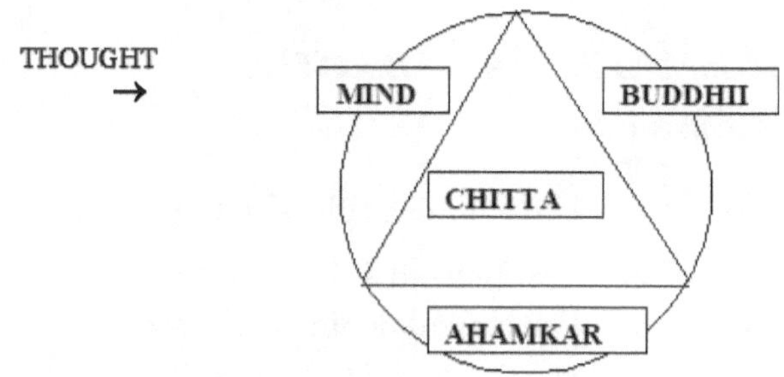

1) **THE MIND \ SENSE ORGANS:** The mind, through sense organs, perceives impressions or sense experience and carries them to Intellect (Buddhi) for distinguishing and classification. The 5 sense organs relate to the five lower energy centers (chakras) which store data, even from past lives.

2) **INTELLECT (BUDDHI):** This faculty discriminates, makes JUDGEMENTAL value, makes distinctions or interpretations accurately or inaccurately. The intellect is Consciousness. Behind Sense organs that classify sensory data, it is evaluating facts and interprets data.

3) **EGO(AHAMKAR):** The Ego maker exists in the lower mercury center. The Ego is what 'I' experience and what 'I' interpret through these experiences. Ego also is a storage bank that interprets particular experiences according to how 'I conceive me'.

The Ego is false self and Atma is true self because all that the entire Ego perceives is transitory, ever changing; when we close off the senses, sensory data disappears only the memory remains and memory changes with time. The atma or spirit on the other hand is unchanging. The Ego is artificial or transitory, for how we see ourselves is based upon our sense experience and judgment of our intellect. The Ego is simply a combination of sense data and the evaluations of that sense data. It is just a thought and a feeling.

An important factor regarding Ego is it is not negative and is not to be destroyed or punished, because without it there cannot be the functioning of human relationship i.e. 'I' and 'You'. It is a necessary evolutionary stage in our total enfoldment. The problem with Ego consciousness is it believes that it is the final reality, because of which the Ego process stops and does not continue in its evolution. The technical term for this process is called ignorance which is the cause of all sufferings.

How Yoga Relates to the Three Factors of Mind-stuff

The Ajna Chakra / 3rd Eye and the Medulla Oblongata /Back 3rd Eye are the manifestations of the individual soul and its full potential. The Spinal Column can be considered a mini Universe. The ascending and the descending energies (Prana and Apana) flowing on the outer surface of the chakras relate to various states of Consciousness. There are certain Yogic techniques which help to purify these two energy channels (Nadi's) opening up the constrictions within the centers of the spinal column. This enables us to lift the currents to the thousand petaled lotus i.e. the Sahasrara which is the symbol of full and total realization of the true self or Atma. In this state of Consciousness lie true joy, love, bliss and wisdom.

However in the pursuit of this evolutionary goal, mankind encounters 2 major obstacles: firstly KARMAS and secondly HIS OWN MENTAL CONDITIONING (memory track).

KARMAS: The first problem is the manifestation of Karma from past. The Karma could be of this birth or lifetimes ago. For further progress on the spiritual path one has to do with or finish off all his past karmas. Through regular practice of the 8 processes of Sai Ashtang Yoga we can break free of this storage of Karma's. Here again immense love for God or Guru and a strong attitude of surrender is a must. Karmas are contained within and around the energy centers of the spinal column. As these karmas are balanced out we move away from these areas and move through the center channel that is the

Sushmna Nadi, freeing the mind-stuff or Consciousness momentarily of past karma emotions and delusions. Our attitude towards life changes positively. This change in attitude becomes a new powerful, positive memory to further spiritual enfoldment.

Karmas exist as vasanas or seed form in the pericarp of the heart of the causal body. Vasana is not Karma but a seed awaiting an appropriate moment to sprout. At the proper moment the causal body releases from its heart these seeds of Karmas that now flow down to the 5 lower chakras i.e. from Vishudha chakra to the Muladhar chakra and back up to the Ajna chakra. After leaving the causal body the seeds circulate in the astral body or mental body becoming caught in the net of various astral chakras. The breath with its inhalation and exhalation creates moisture and heat which causes the seeds to sprout and grow in the astral vehicle or chakras. They then circulate and drop down to the physical body producing Karmic conditions to deal with here in this life time.

Through the practice of sense withdrawal or mind withdrawal, the Yogi draws the Chitta or consciousness from the senses, and thus masters his destiny by withdrawing energy from the Karmas. By breathing through the centre channel or Sushmna Nadi rather than Sun and Moon (Pingala and Ida), heat is generated whereby the Karmic seeds are roasted and burnt up so they cannot sprout, although the Karmic seeds are still released from the causal body to the Physical body.

The heat of the Solar channel or Surya Nadi can never roast the Karmic seeds because the heat is on the outer surface or periphery of your mind/body complex and therefore does not have direct contact with the Karmic seeds, and secondly the heat of the solar channel is not intense enough to roast them.

The second obstacle to man's attainment of self-realization is his own nature —best known as his total memory or conditioning of the mind. Each Chakra has its own consciousness level and because of our past memory, this hinders us from going any where but back to the past. Therefore the average man by his very nature is totally engrossed in the lower Chakras of the spinal column specially the Muladhar, Swadhistan and Manipur levels of consciousness and gets lost in this material world of sense organs. He is involved with such intensity that he identifies himself with mind and body and experiences either pain or pleasures which are temporary.

Pain and pleasure are 2 sides of one coin and cannot be separated. So Yoga or one who practices Yoga attempts to escape from this pleasure and pain principle by pulling away or withdrawing the mind stuff or consciousness from the sense organs. This enables him to lift the life current away from the lower chakras and ascend to the higher chakras.

Both the emotions of pain and pleasure are directly related to the concept of extreme aversion and extreme attraction and they are not suited to a quieted mind, which is necessary to acquire the ability to turn inwards and gain awareness of the higher self in order to obtain depth of wisdom.

So in our daily life we should attempt to detach ourselves from heavy emotionality, because when we become emotional, we are not able to think rightly. This impairs our intellect and consequently the discerning powers. Many extreme aversions and attractions are not always conscious and the mind then interferes with logical patterns.

To start with begin detaching from the more obvious gross objects and then move to detachment from inward and more subtle objects. When we practice detachment we should not be unduly upset with undesirable experiences or get unduly elated with pleasant desirable experiences that manifest.

The Bhagavad Gita points out "Everyone acts according to his own nature against which no effort is ever successful". The nature of the tongue to appreciate taste and sweet taste sweet; be it a householder or a monk. The goal of Yoga is therefore not to change the sense organ but to transcend them.

Just as the tongue is responsible for sense of taste so also are the other organs, for creation of attraction and aversion. Though it is the nature of sense to function they should not be left uncontrolled. The senses need to be guarded and disciplined. We should ever remain completely detached. **Remember, detachment does not mean indifference.**

CONCLUSION: A state of sense withdrawal is attained, when the 5 gross sense organs, the mind and intellect become passive. There should be no misunderstanding that passive or active sense organ means that the sense organs are malfunctioning. The mind has merely pulled away from their force and they have become inactive.

Sense withdrawal is a state of consciousness that is different from the 3 states; every human being experiences i.e. the waking state, the dream state and the dreamless sleep state.

The goal of sense withdrawal or mind withdrawal is valuable because it leads to a fourth state beyond the everyday three, by enabling us to reach into our inner soul, which is known as the Turia State.

What is the Meaning of Sense Withdrawal?

Sense withdrawal is the Yogic technique by which we take the naturally extroverted and outgoing forces of the sense organs and cause them to become introverted and in-turned. This is done by drawing the senses away from their respective objects.

According to Patanjali Yoga Sutra, sense withdrawal occurs when a person disciplines his sense organs to follow his intellect.

Another clear meaning of sense withdrawal is 'Mastery of the senses'. When external objects are present the sense organ cannot recognize them without the command of the mind ex. Sometimes when we are in our own world of thoughts, we do not recognize a friend or a relative who passes by us. When the mind detaches itself from the external objects; sense withdrawal occurs and the sense organs which normally run after external objects cease the running and become stilled. The 5 sense organs being the 5 horses of the chariot of the body guided by the Charioteer- the Mind. Hence when the mind renounces the craving for objects, the sense organs become still.

The keyword is detachment – **not detachment from objects, but detachment from our reactions to these objects** and our sensory perception of the objects.

To get ourselves detached, we should have control of our worldly desires. The practice of **Ceiling on Desires** helps us to control our desires and brings about detachment.

Detachment means detachment from all things. This means detachment towards external as well as internal objects. The common man finds it difficult to release himself from the shackles of worldly objects, and hence he is in bondage or Maya. The bondage results from sense organs, constantly running after objects which produce heavier cravings. Craving just grows and cannot be satisfied.

Unless the mind is completely controlled, sense withdrawal cannot be perfected and without the perfection of sense withdrawal we cannot attain Samadhi, without Samadhi there is no permanent happiness. When sense withdrawal has been mastered, concentration meditation and Samadhi are very easily attained.

The Process of Sense Withdrawal:

Unless the first four gross steps of Yoga are practiced, sense withdrawal is impossible. Pranayama and chanting Mantras are two valuable supports which help in establishing sense withdrawal and gaining control over the life force.

If we control the mind, the senses are controlled. As our breath and thoughts are interlinked; the mind can be controlled by breath control, hence Pranayama. It has been found that as Mantra being more subtle it is difficult to sustain especially when the mind is drawn towards objects. Breathing techniques are more helpful as they are less subtle than mantras. Pranayam enables the mind to let go of what it is attracted to. Once the mind lets go of the object through Pranayam, we may use mantra to go deeper. Pranayam purifies the external gross sense organs and brings them under control. Pranayam has very close connection with the 5 sense organs and thus has a powerful and positive effect on them. This will enable us to go beyond gross sense object into higher states.

Unless we have some degree of mastery over 5 sense organs, it is impossible to understand and attain the 5 subtle organs. And without the understanding of subtle sense organs it is impossible to understand subtle Astral objects such as the Astral Body.

When the intellect is attached to gross objects it is seen that intellect ceases to function in the subtle realm. It is because of the initiation of the intellect the sense organs function. Thus control of the intellect is essential for sense withdrawal. We should train our intellect in such a way that just as the tortoises is able to draw in its limbs so too we should be able to draw in our sense organs.

When we meditate we are slowly moving inward and we slowly start losing our physical body consciousness and hence the external sense organs remain inactive. When a person is in deep meditation, his eyes see nothing, his ears hear nothing, i.e. the senses do not sense anything. During meditation the gross sense organs are nonfunctional and do not acquire any information regarding gross objects. This is so because the mind is inactive. As soon as the mind is free of thoughts or quieted, the gross sense organs cease to have contact with external objects. This total process is called sense-withdrawal or Pratyhara.

Two Types of Sense Withdrawals:

There are two types of Sense Withdrawals namely the gross or physical sense objects which are enjoyed by the gross sense organs and the subtle or astral sense objects, which are enjoyed by the subtle sense organs.

During sense withdrawal; though the mind is inactive, the intellect continues to be active to understand and distinguish. Only the sense organs become inactive and remain calm. During deep meditation, we move inwards in the mental or Astral body, the mind and intellect comes in contact with subtle objects through subtle or astral sense organs. These subtle astral objects can only be perceived and thus enjoyed. These astral objects are of great beauty and attraction; there are chances that we get attached to them and do not progress towards our goal. Hence sense withdrawal of even these subtle or astral sense objects should be attained.

Unless both these levels are mastered, only then the Yogi enters the super-subtle realm and its super- subtle objects. Herein lies Samadhi. Sense withdrawal cannot be complete until the intellect is completely divested of all its attachment to gross and subtle objects.

There Are Four Stages of Sense Control or Sense Withdrawal

1) **Progressive Detachment (Yatamana): Love and Hate** are the two extremely powerful emotions that are deeply ingrained in human consciousness and pull us towards given objects. It is not only the love emotion that draws us towards an object but hate also drives the mind and holds us to that object of hate. Hence these two powerful emotions are to be dealt with, which is the first stage of progressive detachment.

   Because of selfish possessive love, people experience grief. With the help of intellect, by right understanding and utilization of sense withdrawal these 2 emotions of love and hate can be controlled and craving is softened by withdrawing the senses from these two mental emotions. Pure Love or Prema, is unselfish or selfless love that is divine and only such love can confer true happiness, bliss and peace.

2) **Exclusive Detachment (Vyatireka):** We have to be aware and observe life in general along with our own life, clearly recognizing and understanding the negativity that exists in various objects especially the ever changing and nonpermanance of these objects. Only then will we be able to perceive how mankind suffers because of its attachment to those objects and not because of an innate negativity within the object itself. (ex. air conditioner or any artistic picture). When we perceive the dangers and negatives within certain objects, we will be able to decide and determine which objects are detrimental to our own life style. This can be done by determination and understanding which of the negatives have been renounced and insuring that they stay renounced and which are yet to be renounced.

   An easy way of doing this is by preparing a list of negatives from which you want to detach. Put them in priority order and follow our plan to attain proper harmonizing renunciation. This is what exclusive detachment implies.

3) **One Organ Detachment (Eka-indriya):** In our dealing with relationships in our day to day life we persistently indulge in emotionalities. The residue of these emotional forces enters into the depths of our memory bank in the chakras. This has a very deep unconscious interfering effect on the functioning of the intellect. The activation of a given sense organ depends

on how deeply and frequently the emotion has created the impression upon the mind stuff or consciousness ex. If some film magazines and novels are given away as trash, we would not be much upset. But if we see Bhagavad Gita (a highly revered scripture) given in the trash we would definitely be upset. The word Bhagavad Gita has made much deeper emotional impression on our sub-conscious mind than the other magazines and novels.

By practicing the technique of detaching ourselves from one single organ, all day long, each day of our life, the Yogi assures that these interferences do not take place. We should refrain from emotionality. All the sense organs should be well controlled; only then we can attain sense withdrawal or higher stages of yoga.

The first stage is concerned with people and personalities.

The second stage is concerned with objects surrounding us. i.e. our happiness should not be determined by objects.

The third relates more to our inner dreams and spiritual enfoldment plans. These are not depending on gross objects but yet they must be renounced so that we find our happiness and wisdom along our pathway of life.

Remember; the cause of unhappiness is our attitude and our attachment to objects, not to the innate quality of objects.

4) **Controlled Detachment (Vashikarana):** After practicing the above 3 stages extensively, we reach a fourth stage in which deep buried innate impressions do not arise and disturb the intellect, and no matter which object, gross or subtle, is presented before us, we are not disturbed. Thus controlled detachment is acquired and detachment becomes an every day part of life.

Sense Withdrawal Techniques:

Neti or Negation Technique:

This is an important technique by practicing which we attain sense-withdrawal from gross and subtle objects. It helps us in detaching ourselves from all objects. This technique breaks the illusion that we are the body and the mind.

Sit comfortably in a meditative posture. Close the eyes and turn inward. The place we sit should be quiet and pleasant, comfortable without physical or emotional distractions. The temperature of the room should be comfortable. The time of the practice each day should be the same, very early in the morning or late in the evening. Keep the spine straight. Sit on a folded blanket with the body at full attention without tension. The body must remain perfectly motionless.

Now begin, taking a deep breath and relax. Be completely aware, without any physical or mental tension. Let the thoughts flow. Watch them without judgment…. Just watch them. Be one with self. Watch the thoughts unconcernedly. Try not to join one thought with the other or do not form a chain of thoughts. Be mindful of what is happening in the inward universe…. Meet the mind. As we are mindful of the thoughts, as we see a thought, mentally think and mentally feel it: Neti, neti, neti. This means 'I' am not this thought. I am not that thought; I am not thought at all' In essence we experience an important realization: I am not this thought that I see, nor am I this thought watching that thought…. I am not the thought at all.

As we do not identify ourselves with the stream of thoughts, we begin to realize that we are not the mind but the real self. This process is so simple to describe yet so difficult to perform. But practice makes the person perfect. Hence it is important to master this technique. This technique should be practiced 3 to 7 minutes a day. It would be helpful to practice it for the rest of your life. We will, however, find major benefits within weeks, if not days.

The Yoni Mudra:

Another technique for attaining sense withdrawal. It is extremely important for it astralizes your consciousness and helps you to move to subtler realms.

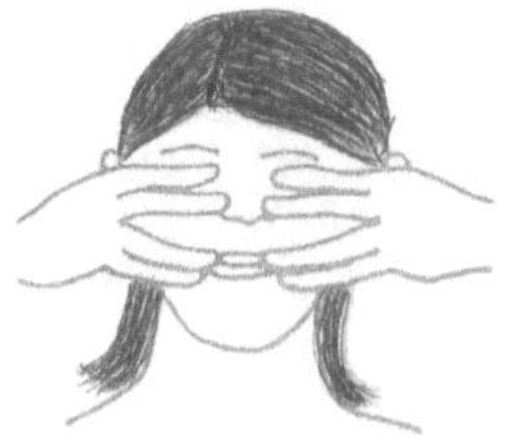

Diagram of Yoni Mudra:

Sit erect, with spine straight, resting the elbows on the table or some small support. The support should be of a perfect height so that we can place our thumbs on our ears without slumping forward or straining upward. Place the thumbs comfortably but tightly on each of the tragus so that they close the openings of the ears. The eyes are closed and focused at the root of the nose at the eyebrows. The index fingers are placed below the eyes to hold them firmly. They are pressed lightly as to prevent movement of the eyeballs, assisting the eye hold at the Ajna chakra. Each middle finger rests gently on the nasal passages; the ring fingers are placed on the upper lip and little fingers on the lower lip. Now take a deep breath, hold and press the fingers so that all the sense organs are stopped. This is known as Yoni Mudra.

Take a slow and a deep breath, hold the breath. While holding our breath comfortably, mentally turn inward, with such intensity that we forget the whole external universe. This is sense withdrawal. Full attention is focused on the Ajna chakra, looking for and perceiving the light that is literally there. At first, most people perceive only darkness. Later, it appears to be a circular darkness at the sun center. Without straining, continue to look. Later, a hazy circular egg-shaped light will appear. Still later a circle of light can be seen. This circle of light then takes on various colorations; gold, then blue.

When the breath can no longer be comfortably held, release all the fingers. Exhale slowly. Inhale slowly, hold again, turning yet deeper inward. This technique helps us to control the senses and also to concentrate at the 3rd eye.

We have just studied how the four outer gross steps help us to establish mind control. When mind is controlled, the senses are naturally controlled. When sense withdrawal is established it becomes easy to concentrate and so now we will discuss Dharana or concentration in our next Chapter.

SAI RAM

Chapter VI

Dharana or Concentration

Yama, Niyama, Asana and Pranayama are the 4 outer limbs or stages of Yoga while Sense Withdrawal, concentration, meditation and Samadhi are called the inner limbs or stages.

As Sense Withdrawal or Pratyahara is mastered, concentration begins. As concentration is finally mastered, meditation commences. Following this, Samadhi slowly manifests. The timing of beginning and ending of each stage cannot be said or measured. These separate movements occur simultaneously with eminent speed when one sits for the practice of silent sitting. It is for purpose of explanation that we break down Yoga into parts.

The ancient texts state that when we hold our mind on any given gross object for 12 seconds with no distraction whatsoever, we have technically attained concentration. In those 12 seconds the mind may not be interrupted by any internal or external secondary thought whatsoever. If 144 seconds i.e.2 minutes and 24 seconds of concentration are attained, then we will slowly glide into meditation. This is effortless holding of the object in the mind. If 1,728 seconds of meditation (or 29 minutes) are sustained a state of Samadhi is reached. If Samadhi can be held for 48 minutes (a muhurta) Liberation (Kaivalya) is attained. This mathematical calculation is based upon information in the Kurma Purana.

Concentration, meditation and Samadhi is a single continuous process and the three together is called Samyama in Sanskrit. It means holding Consciousness together. This is a combined effort of all the three with a dynamic thrust which is inward and upward in order to explore and understand the nature of Consciousness, and ultimately transcend it.

The above three, that is concentration, meditation and Samadhi are mental operations and not of the physical body and therefore described as inner limbs. They are connected with subtle internal mind actions and therefore this is called the Yoga of spiritual action.

When the mind is free from distraction, concentration is performed. So, just as we can learn to swim by actually going into the waters and doing the specific action of swimming and not by just sitting and thinking of swimming so to we can learn to free our mind from distraction by trying to concentrate. Merely thinking becomes a distraction to learning. So a distracted mind cannot learn to concentrate and without concentration we can never truly free the mind. Just as gold ore is purified by heating it in a crucible, so too the mind is purified by placing it in the crucible of concentration. Concentration is the crucible of controlled, determined thinking.

Concentration is not a mental condition but a function of the mind. We can compare concentration with driving or walking. Driving or walking is not a condition within which we find yourself but a function we perform in order to travel somewhere. The same concept applies to meditation and Samadhi.

TYPES OF DHARANA

Broadly speaking there are two types of Dharana or concentration:

- **Baaya Dharana:** Something done outside which goes inwards ex. The Mantra chanted consciously then the same chanting is continued by the mind unknowingly.

  This is the highest type of Dharana. Outward Dharana turns to inward Dharana. Phonetic chanting leading silent mental chanting is known as MANTRA YOGA.

- **Antar Dharana:** Gazing or seeing the idol till the image can be clearly seen by the mental eye.

Controlling the Mind

From the ultimate Pure Consciousness descends the Prakrurti or Shakti or Energy.

From this Energy descends the Trigunas namely the Sattva, the calm equanimity state or state of compassion, Rajas, the overactive or hyper activity state and Tamas, the dull or lethargic state. These three have their hold on the mind.

These trigunas have an evolutionary process. The mind is first dull and then moves away from lethargy, becomes passionate. In passionate state it becomes hyperactive and runs wild and yet it is higher than no action at all. Then the mind rebalances and becomes compassionate and attains equipoise. This is the highest state.

These three qualities play a very important role on the physical as well as mental level of all human beings and therefore we find an average man to be dull and lethargic at one point and compassionate and wise at the next moment. This cycle keeps on repeating itself and yet independent of these interactions there is a basic continual state of consciousness that prevails. Therefore we find that sometimes a person is lethargic, passionate, hyperactive or serene.

- When the mind is overcome by dullness or Tamas it lacks the power to differentiate between wisdom and foolishness.

- When the mind is overcome by hyper activity i.e Rajas, the person becomes more ambitious and is always discontented. This hyper activity and ambition gives rise to more and more desires and when desires are fulfilled he craves for more and when they are not fulfilled, he is frustrated. All this gives rise to feverish unrest and irresistible cravings. This being a never- ending vicious circle, man gets trapped in his own self created trap. He becomes more and more entangled in the worldly superficiality of life.

- When mind is ruled by equanimity i.e. Sattva, it unfolds, and is collected, serene and wise. This is a state needed for the attainment of spiritual insight. Through concentration, this is attained.

The modern day's hectic schedules have put most human beings out of balance with life. Because of this imbalance there is disharmony, which causes mind to be scattered and dull. So the best remedy is concentration, which is best suited for centering and rebalancing the equilibrium of the mind stuff or consciousness.

In Bhagavad Gita, Sri Krishna points out the necessity for equilibrium saying: 'Arjuna, the practice of Yoga is not for him who eats too much or too little; not is it for him who sleeps too much or keeps awake excessively. He who moderates his eating, his work, his recreation, his sleep, he alone is capable of mastering Yoga'.

The concerted effort to remove the physical and mental imbalances of your lifestyle begins with the practice of concentration. This effort is reciprocal, for as you learn to concentrate and gain success in Yoga, your life will become more balanced and meaningful. However it is necessary to remove the impediments to concentration.

Obstacles to Concentration

There are a few impediments to the practice of concentration and the student should be watchful so as to overcome them.

1) Uncontrolled emotions and attachments are a major obstacle to learning concentration. So learn to control your emotions and cravings as you move through life.

2) Hectic and heavy daily work schedules may make it difficult to find time and energy to practice concentration. Priority should be given to this important practice and some energy and time must be spared for this activity.

3) Extreme physical and mental weakness will impair your ability to learn concentration. This will not prohibit you from learning but will definitely retard your process. So to keep yourself fit you should regularly practice postures i.e. Asanas and breath control i.e. Pranayama.

4) Concentration is not only important in your spiritual life but also in the psycho-bio- mental functioning of your individual being. Lack of

intuitional understanding of the importance of concentration will keep you away from the goal.

5) Simply perform the exercise of concentration quietly and consistently without thought of how well you are doing. You will be surprised at your rapid progress. Too much analyzing and concern over gain or loss in the mastery of concentration will seriously jeopardize your enfoldment.

6) Proper attitude towards the mind is required for your progress. Always remind yourself on all levels of your being, of this important psychological concept 'I am not the mind. I have a mind and a body, but they are merely instruments for my expression. I am the self-existent one or the soul or atma or Pure Consciousness.

THEORY OF THE MIND-AS PER YOGA

The word concentration comes from a Latin word, which means one-pointedness. Concentration means the ability to direct the mind and maintain a full and exclusive attention on the object of concentration. When the state of concentration is mastered, then the ability to stop the mind and look back at the passing thoughts or thinking itself occurs. As per Yoga, concentration is a practicing technique; by practicing regularly you gain conscious control over your mental faculties.

Concentration is a natural in-built ability man possesses, but it is involuntary and uncontrolled. It is the result of the power and forces the sense organs have over the mind. When you are able to hold to the state of concentration as long as the related task demands, you are said to be concentrating. You should be able to concentrate consciously upon whatever the mind wills.

Concentration also means, the mind should be able to let go of the state of concentration when the related task is over. It means that the mind should be disciplined to let go when required ex. problem solving. The mind must be focused on problem solving only till it is solved and must not keep on brooding and thinking about the problem all the time. You and your mind should be able to let go once the problem is solved.

When you practice concentration regularly and are able to hold your mind, the scattered energies are gathered together and work like the search light removing the darkness and enabling you to perceive into the distance.

Only when the mind and intellect is used, undisturbed by distracting emotions and cravings or desires, can you free yourself and achieve the goal you have set in this lifetime ex. In the epic of Mahabharat, Arjuna aiming the wooden fish eye is a very good example of focused concentration. You should be able to close out all disruptive and irrelevant awareness if you have to hit the mark.

In short Dharana means a mind which is withdrawn, and focused on one point. It can be put on one thought i.e. Mantra, or Pratik, or Murti or on thought.

By closing our 5 channels and concentrating through one track, we bring in the power to bear on any one of the items mentioned above.

Thought becomes very powerful.

The Function of Concentration:

The function of concentration is to focus the mind, which like a search light, gives it the power to pay attention or focus attention to the object of concentration. The object is first imagined and then focused upon. Secondly shift the object of concentration to the mind itself which itself is a state of consciousness. Thirdly, be a witness to the mind as a separate entity. After you are able to witness it for quite some time, acquire interest in Pure Consciousness because you, as witness, is none other than the Pure Consciousness itself.

As concentration itself means to hold or focus the mind on one object only, there is self restriction. This self restriction is necessary in order to finally transcend the thought itself and not the object. This happens when you concentrate one-pointedly; slowly your thoughts reduce and you then transcend the thought.

Distinction Between Concentration and Meditation:

1) A major distinction between concentration and Meditation is that concentration is self restricted state of mind which is held with great effort. Meditation is the effortless holding of the mind to its object with a feeling of expansiveness which is referred to by the western psychologists as unrestricted free association. In Yoga it is called the stream of Consciousness.

2) The process of concentration is effortless and without any tensing or forcing. It is a calm, intense and directed activity of the mind. When you practice concentration and meditation, all the fancy thoughts, imaginative thinking, day dreaming etc. should not be confused with concentration. There should be focused attention and complete awareness of the mind without any tension while concentrating and meditating.

Concentration Procedure

1) Concentration is holding the mind to a single object, simple or complex, large or small, concrete or abstract. Ex. A beautiful rose, just a dot or any God or Guru's image or photo etc.

2) Concentrating on the image of your Guru or God will be more helpful for future meditation.

3) Initially when you start the practice of concentration, you may require repeating a mantra or creating a mental picture of a particular image in order to keep your mind on the object of concentration.

4) After many practice sessions, you firmly establish yourself after which you will not feel the need for repeating of the mantra or any mental image. You will thus be able to gently control the mind and learn to induce a mood.

5) When you have truly learned concentration, inducing the mood of the object will become automatic and you will have no need to visualize it. The object of concentration is held by the mind itself.

This is Called Contemplation.

Practice of Concentration

Sit in any comfortable meditative posture. Gently try to visualize the form of your Guru\God or any concrete object. Try to draw your mind to its simple physical anatomy, the hair, the eyes, the face, dress to the feet etc. You may then move to its subtler qualities such as the way he talks, walks, expressions, movements etc. With control but without tension, you draw from concentration all that you can relate to God.

In order to understand the object of concentration you may use the 7 interrogative pronouns, Who? What? Where? How? Which? Why? And When? Ask simple questions about the object of concentration ex. Who is this? Give a pause, waiting for some answer. Then ask the second question What is this? so on and so forth.

The above 7 interrogative technique for concentration is a way to extract data and information as well as concentrating the mind. In future this helps you to have communication and guidance from your real self or your Guru. When you are learning to concentrate, you may have to return again and again to your object of concentration, for an extended period of time, as the fickleness of our monkey mind does not allow it to be steady so very easily.

3 Important Points for Controlled Thinking | Yogic Concentration

1) The mind by its very nature is very fickle and keeps jumping from one thought to another. Hence this monkey mind keeps on wandering. When the mind wanders one must not get upset or angry. This will destroy your concentration without reproach, draw the mind back and reunite it with the object of concentration. Continue doing so till the mind realizes it is much easier to hold on to the object of concentration rather than wander elsewhere. Concentration begins when the mind of its own volition holds to what you are concentrating on, without any heavy aberration Ex……. Riding a horse

Initially when you start practicing concentration the mind wanders very frequently and you have to draw it back again and again to the object of concentration. After 6 months of regular practice, the wandering reduces; after about a year it will wander 10 to 15 times and in about 2 to 3 years it may not wander at all but remain completely fixed on the object of concentration.

2) The second important point while concentrating is that you should not engage in tangential thinking which will lead you away from the object of concentration.

   Ex. If you are concentrating on your God or Guru, do not hold to the thoughts of other people around Him or you will miss the concentration. If you are concentrating on your God or Guru, hold your complete awareness and attention on your God or Guru, with the understanding fully that you are attempting to isolate Him from the rest of the universe. In actuality this cannot be done but the effort to do so will help you to separate your own consciousness from the matrix of your thoughts and emotions. This is a very powerful yogic technique and in doing so you will gain insight into your consciousness.

3) The third point of Yogic concentration or controlled thinking is, you should not confuse tangential thinking with the mode of return. This is a subtle point. Ex. If you are concentrating on your God and Guru and if the mode of return has risen then this may lead to thoughts of how He walks, talks ….and further how He has been guiding you and others…. and how He has been doing a lot of social projects….. and again having loving and thoughts of gratitude for Him. Here you have deviated from the object of concentration, but that diversion has led you to return to the object of concentration and therefore you have completed a cycle. Your mode of return automatically returns you to the point where it began. When the mode of return arises, concentration has been mastered. The completion of a cycle has a very symbolic significance. At this stage concentration has been attained and you have slipped over to the next stage of meditation. With a little practice this mode of return can be induced at will.

POINTS TO MAKE YOUR CONCENTRATION POWERFUL

When you follow Yogic principles that is Yama, Niyam, Pranayama, asana etc. and adjust your daily lifestyle by removing all mental and physical imbalances in your life and add serenity of your mind and then concentration will be easy and well focused.

Given below are some of the points which will help you to make your concentration powerful.

1) **Follow Ceiling on Desires**. This will help you to curtain unnecessary wants and desires, control your craving and eliminate unwanted superficial wants. Not all your needs and wants ought to be discarded.

2) Try to keep your state of mind calm and peaceful throughout the day and not only while concentrating.

3) Limit your day-to-day activities to those most significant. By doing so you will have more time and improve your concentration, life style, reduce your stress level and have longevity.

4) When you practice breathing exercise it will be easy for you to breathe more deeply. This will help you to reduce your thoughts.

5) Effort should be made to remain happy, cheerful and friendly.

6) Self introspection is an very important part of your life, especially when you are practicing concentration and living your day to day life. Always be mindful. This develops greater perception and greater intuition.

Guidelines to Practicing Concentration

1) Find a comfortable **place** where daily you can sit and concentrate without disturbance. The same area or place should not be used for any other purpose or even to practice yogic asana because the vibrations are different and are contradictory to the vibrations needed for concentration.

2) Choose the best **time**, early or late in the day for concentration. Concentrate at that fixed time. The best timing is 4a.m. to 8 a.m. in the morning and 4p.m. to 8 p.m. in the evening as they are called Brahmamurat.

3) **Asana**: Use a meditation mat made of wool or flannel. This too should not be used for any other purpose. As far as possible this mat should not be washed or touched by any other person as it carries very powerful vibrations which are a very good support for concentration. Hence preserve it well, so that it remains clean and no other person touches it.

4) **Procedure** for beginning concentration.
   a) Sit in any comfortable Asana or posture.
   b) Eyes closed focus on the trikuti or between the eyebrows.
   c) Take a deep breath and relax.
   d) Chant OM aloud slowly 3 times.
   e) Practice Pranayama for a few moments.
   f) Prayer to your God or Guru.
   g) Proceed to focus on the object of concentration.
   These 7 steps will drive away the external fields and relax the body and quiet the mind.

5) Begin concentration on gross objects or the image of your God and Guru and later on subtler objects. Regularity in concentration is more important than the choice of the object.

6) When you are in deep concentration you are not aware of your external surroundings and there is no perception of body awareness or body consciousness.

7) In the beginning practices your mind will run wild and you may feel you are being disturbed by more thoughts than normal. This is a very natural thing to happen. You may have to treat the mind like a child and bring it lovingly back to the object of concentration repeatedly by giving it directions, till it settles down.

8) Gently settle down, eyes closed, relaxed and concentrate and be serene in your practice of concentration, or else you will not find enjoyment in the technique. And if there is no enjoyment; your mind will not be prepared to return to the practice of concentration.

9) With constant introspection and self analysis keep a check on the mind and be sure that it is not involved in day dreaming or jumping from one thought to another.

10) While concentrating, if there are disturbing thoughts or if the mind is restless and you feel you are losing your concentration then without getting upset or angry, very gently return the mind back to the object of concentration. Any forceful movement will destroy your concentration. Unfortunately most of time, the beginners make this mistake of wrestling with the mind.

11) When the person who is ready for the practice of concentration is not completely relaxed, he feels the need to urinate. This is caused by an irritation in the micturition center of the spinal cord. This is an indication that he needs to relax more and become calmer before starting concentration.

Techniques to Help Concentration

VISUALIZATION TECHNIQUE: Creating a personal Meditation Room

Just as we have kitchen for cooking, bedroom for sleeping etc. We can **mentally create** our personal meditation room.

Benefits:

1) In big cities, it is difficult to have a separate meditation room, hence this mental creation.

2) We create a serene and peaceful environment by creating a meditation room.

3) There is a drastic change in the **Mental Vibration** because you meditate in that atmosphere and environment regularly.

4) When you travel or go outstation; you can still meditate in the same peaceful atmosphere because it is a mental creation.

5) If you feel you are bored with this meditation room, you may create a new meditation room.

How to Create the Meditation Room

Sit straight with your spine erect but very comfortably. Close your eyes and focus at the 3rd eye or Ajna Chakra.

Mentally visualize a beautiful room as your personal meditation room. This room can be **created anyw here** on earth, sea, sky, mountains, forest etc. where you feel at peace and comfortable.

Decorate it as per your choice and colour of the room, curtains etc. As this is a meditation room it has **no furniture, except 1) A chair for your God or Guru to sit. 2) A lamp to be lit. 3) Dim lighting, but you can see everything clearly. 4) Your fixed place and fix asana to sit.**

You may decorate the **wall with Photos or Paintings, Rangoli or Flower decoration etc.**

Mentally, enter the meditation room; light the lamp, incense or agarbatti (optional). Sit on your asana and start with the daily process of Meditation.

Concentration Gazing:

Definition: Concentration is defined as 'an intense, calm, watching, accompanied by attention of the mind without tension'

2 Basic guidelines are:

a) The eyes may be either opened or closed. However it is recommended that eyes be closed for deeper concentration.

b) There are four focal points of concentration, and one can focus on any one of the points as per the suitability of the person. The four focal points are the root of the nose rightly known as the trikuti or the Ajna Chakra; the tip of the nose; the heart or the Anahat Chakra, and lastly the length of the spinal cord.

The Ajna Chakra and the Anahat Chakra are the two most important points.

FRONTAL GAZE: (Bhrumadhya drishti): In the frontal gaze the attention is focused at the 3rd eye or Ajna Chakra. This is at the root of the nose between the eyebrows. Sit in the meditative posture, close your eyes and gently focus at the trikuti. Do not stare. Just gently gaze. There is no violent effort involved in this procedure. Hold your attention as long as you are comfortable and then gradually increase the duration of concentration. The frontal gaze must always be performed with eyes closed.

There is a mention of this concentration technique in the Bhagvad Geeta Chapter 6. This technique is very commonly used by most meditation practitioners. The mind is easier to control when you practice this technique.

- **NASAL GAZE: (Nasikagra-drishti)** Concentrate on the tip of the nose with eyes open or half open but start with eyes closed. This practice is described in the Bhagwat Geeta, chapter VI, shloka 13 and this practice rapidly steadies and deepens the power of concentration.

- **HEART GAZE: (Anahat-dristi)** Concentrate on the Heart or Anahat Chakra with eyes closed. This gaze is utilized by devotional yogis. This gaze is recommended for practitioners with devotional nature. There are practitioners who focus on both the Ajna and Anahat chakra to join the connection between the head and the heart.

- **SPINAL GAZE:** Close the eyes and focus on the totality of your spinal column. In this technique you are to simultaneously see with your mind's eye and to feel the entire (Shusumna) or balanced center channel. This gaze is used by the Hatha Yogis, Kundalini Yogis and some Kriya Yogis. A balanced state of consciousness evolves from this technique. It is an extremely difficult to perform for beginners. So beginners are advised to focus on smaller areas like the trikuti.

- **AUDIO TECHNIQUE OR THE TICKING EXERCISE:** Sit in any meditative posture. Set a watch or clock close to you so that you can hear the ticking sound. Close the eyes and perform frontal gaze (Trikuti), concentrating on the ticking sound. Hold to this sound to the exclusion of all other sounds, thoughts or feelings. See how long your mind is able to remain fixed on this sound. Repeat daily. This can also be done with music.

- **VISUAL TECHNIQUE OR THE 'WHO AM I' EXERCISE:** It is difficult for an average person to penetrate the inner mind much less the origin of consciousness. However, we must start somewhere into this investigation of consciousness. The starting point is the exploration of the mind itself. During this exploration you realize you are one thing and your mind another thing. Here is the greatest concentration technique there is.

Form a meditative pose utilizing frontal gaze (trikuti) with eyes closed. Employ the 7 interrogative pronoun technique mentioned earlier and repeatedly keep asking yourself, **Who** am I…..? **What** am I….? **Where** am I…..? **Why** am I ……..? **Which** one am I ……? **When** am I…..? **How** am I…..? When you have finished the first round, return to them, asking the same. When you practice this regularly, you will attain deeper concentration and also insight into your own nature.

- **TRATAK:** is one of the methods to increase the power of concentration. There are many types of Tratak but the **POINT TRATAK** is a better and easier to practice.

- **POINT TRATAK:** Put a black dot on a large art paper. Affix it on the wall opposite. Squat at a location two or three feet away from the wall. Now fix your eyes on the black dot without winking your eyes.

After some time the practitioner will see the dot moving in various direction on the paper, and sometimes it may vanish. At a particular stage the practitioner will not see the black dot. Instead a dazzling light will seem to have replaced the black dot. When you see a thing like this, take it that your efforts have been crowned with success.

Now introduce a change in the practice. Draw a circle around the black dot in black colour. Now, once again, fix your eye on the black dot. Gradually the practitioner will see that the black circle has vanished. It has been replaced with brilliant lines sprouting about. Again it is an indication of your success as a practitioner.

Introduce another change. Draw seven similar lines around the black dot. Ensure that the black dot remains at the centre of the lines. Now fix your eyes on the black dot. Gradually the practitioner will begin to feel that the black dot as also one or two circumferences does not seem to be present at the same location. As he goes ahead with the practice he will find that all seven circles have disappeared. It means you have already entered your **Turiyawastha. - The most engrossing state of spiritual trance.** It is a delightful state because the seven lines disappear only when your own inner light blazes forth. The inner splendor gets reflected on the paper with such extraordinary power that the black dot and the black circumferences around the black dot do not appear to exist. The brilliant golden light which you find in its place is nothing but your own inner light which, having been reflected on the paper, lets into your eyes. This is said to be an outstanding achievement.

The same can be practiced with 1" dot and 7 circumferences. When you reach the above level, you can see and hear objects from far away etc. But here our main purpose is to have deeper concentration and not the power of clairvoyance. **With such powerful concentration it is easy to slowly glide into Meditation or DHYANA. How this is done, we will explore in our next Chapter of Dhyana.**

SAI RAM

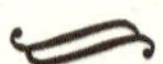

Chapter VII
Meditation or Dhyana

Having covered the first two of the inner stages of Sense withdrawal and concentration, we now come to the seventh state of Sai Astang Yoga called meditation.

When one sustains and maintains the focus of attention through Dharana unbound by time and space, it becomes Dhyana (Meditation). Deep concentration destroys the Rajas and Tamas Gunas of the mind and develops the Satvika gunas (qualities).

Man is born and reborn because of his endless desires. To fulfill these desires, he has to perform actions. Actions are of two types, the ones which are binding and the other actions which are liberating. **The binding actions** are actions related to external object, where there is an expectation of results. This expectation leads to craving and greed while further they lead to Ahamkar or 'I' and Mamakar or 'Mine'. These actions keep man in bondage or Maya or Illusion and he keeps traveling round and round in the cycle of birth and death.

The liberating actions are those actions which are pure and selfless. Even when functioning in the day-to-day worldly activities, if one has no expectations of the result, and offers all his actions at the Divine Lotus Feet of the Lord at the end of each day with the understanding that he is not the doer but only an instrument in the Lord's hand then he can be free from the feelings of 'I' and 'Mine', craving and greed. Such actions are mentioned in the Bhagvad Geeta as **Nishkama Karma**. By the practice of such actions, one will automatically practice the 'Niyama' (the second step of Sai Astang Yoga, which is observance of Satya, Dharma, Shanti, Prema and Ahimsa).

While practicing the above selfless actions, if we practices **Namasmarana** or continuous chanting of the Lord's name, this will help to tame the mad monkey mind. This practice will also be helpful to perform right and selfless actions. The best way to perform selfless action is Meditation or Dhyana.

Practicing Yama and Niyama (given the earlier Chapters) and by continuous repetition of the Lord's name (Japa) will bring purity of mind, and the mind and intelligence will be cleansed and tamed to concentrate (Dharana) and thus be prepared for Meditation.

God has endowed man with unlimited powers of which he is unaware. To get back this awareness of the powers we must make use of the instruments of repetition of Lord's name or Japa and Meditation. What is the use if one has a car but does not know how to drive it? So each one of us should be aware of these powers within and utilize them to seek and understand the ultimate Universal Consciousness or God, which is the very base of the entire creation.

There are three fundamental basic requirements for an aspirant or disciple to reach the goal of self realization. They are

1) **Immense love for God**
2) **Purity of mind**
3) **Attitude of complete self surrender.**

With these three powerful tools, one is very much inspired to sit for the practice of meditation which is most required especially in the initial stages.

WHAT IS MEDITATION?

Meditation is a process or a function of treading the inward path to reach the destination of the Real Self (Self Realization) for which the mind is trained to Concentrate (Dharana). Meditation cannot be taught, it happens. We start with concentration. We can concentrate on any beautiful object which evokes the feeling of contentment, but it is highly advisable to concentrate on the image of our God or Guru together with the Japa.

People who believe that chanting the Lord's name and meditation will help them to get worldly desires satisfied, are totally mistaken. Meditation and Japa or chanting the name of the Lord are for focusing on the Lord with **one-pointed attention,** so that the mind can be steady and not wander in all direction. The mind can thus be trained to focus inward on the Lord which means concentration or Dharana, and not get distracted on impermanent sensory objects.

When one is able to focus with **one-pointed attention**, the mind is said to be Contemplating. During contemplation the mind slowly glides into meditation. So meditation happens. Hence Concentration or Dharana means holding one subtle object with effort and Meditation or Dhyana means holding effortlessly, one subtle object and calm, deep quietude of the mind. The calmness of the mind is the link between meditation and Samadhi, where thought is transcended and you ascend towards spiritual consciousness.

The timing of beginning and ending of the process of Concentration, Contemplation and meditation cannot be measured or mentioned. They are separate movements occurring or happening simultaneously with eminent speed when one sits for the practice of silent sitting. It is for the purpose of understanding and explanation they are divided into parts in Yoga. Therefore Concentration i.e. Dharana, Meditation i.e. Dhyana and Samadhi or Equipoise, always function together to form a sequence. This single operation is called **Samyama.**

Types of Meditation

There are two types of meditations, **a) Gross or Stul Upasana or meditation. b) Subtle or Sukshma or Nirguna Upanasa or meditation.**

a) **Gross or Stul or Saguna meditation:** We start concentration by focusing on an image of idol (imagining mentally). In the beginning it is not easy to focus as our mind keeps on wandering because of its very nature. So when the mental modifications of Sankalpa, Vikalpa (i.e to do or not to do) stops, the flow of the thoughts reduces and finally the mind becomes steady. When the mind is steady, like constant flow of oil or like a flame which is straight and steady then we may say that meditation has happened.

b) **Subtle or Sukshma Nirguna meditation:** When one has reached the above state, one slowly shifts to the subtle state where there is no image or idol, only the feeling. As there is no image or idol and only a subtle feeling, it is said to be Nirguna meditation. By regular and constant practice of this meditation one can attain the ultimate fruits of the Sadhana i.e. Moksha or self- Realization.

Obstacles During the Practice of Meditation

1) The nature of the mind being fickle, it keeps on jumping from one thought to another. We have to train the mind to sit quietly at one place and at a fixed time. Usually it is said that it takes 21 days for the mind to get habituated. So initially beginners in this practice will find it a bit difficult, but we should sit for the practice with strong will and determination and win over the mind. Once the mind gets habituated to the time, surprisingly it reminds you of the same. So be committed to yourself and practice meditation regularly.

2) If we are careless, inattentive, negligent and unconcerned about the internal and external conditions of life, there are chances of missing some important experiences in meditation and also the changes that take place in our internal and external life.

3) Any sort of physical and/or mental illness could be a great obstacle to meditation. Hence the outer stages of yoga – Yama, Niyama, Asanas and Prananyama are given importance to ensure physical and mental fitness.

4) Sometimes, due to circumstances in the external life, we may feel dullness and laziness due to which the mind and body are inactive. Do we stop our routine activities of brushing our teeth, eating etc. when we feel lazy? No. Similarly make meditation a part of your routine activity.

The Process and Different States in Meditation

1) **Concentration:** The first state is concentration. When we sit comfortably in the meditative pose, with eyes closed and our focus at the Ajna chakra or the 3rd eye center and try to concentrate on the object of concentration, the very first thing we will observe is that there is a continuous and steady flow of thoughts. These thoughts are about our day to day life. The mind will definitely try to put obstacles by bringing in unnecessary thoughts. We should not give up. But slowly as we try to focus on the object of concentration, then thoughts linked to this object will start flowing. Ex. If the object of concentration is the image of our God or Guru, then thoughts pertain to Him will start flowing. If for some reason this does not happen then we should consciously start thinking about our God or Guru so that only such thoughts flow. The flow of the thought is so rapid that it is difficult to distinguish between one thought and the other. Thus the process of concentration has started.

2) **Contemplation:** In this second state we become aware that we are the observer and we are not the mind but the observer observing the thought process. We start watching our thoughts. Just be a witness and observe the thoughts. Do not be JUDGEMENTAL or criticize or get disturbed by these thoughts. Only witness them without joining one thought to another, or do not "chain" your thoughts. Slowly the thoughts start reducing and we become aware of the gaps between the two thoughts. These gaps keep on widening and then the thoughts are slowly reduced to three, two and then one thought about the object of meditation so that we can say there is complete one-pointedness on the object of meditation. When we achieve one pointedness we start contemplation that is be focused on the one thought on the one object of concentration.

3) **Meditation:** Meditation happens as we are contemplating on the one thought and one image. We start becoming aware of the void (the feeling we get in the gap between the two thoughts). This process of awareness of the void and awareness of the one thought and one object continues for some time till we move deeper within and the meditation becomes deeper.

4) **Deep Meditation:** When we move still deeper in meditation, we are more centered in the feeling of the void or the gap than the one thought and one image. At this stage there is no thought and no image, only the feeling-state, the feeling of the void or nothingness. Our awareness has gone beyond the thinking process and therefore beyond thought or mind. This is deep meditation.

Within void exists the feeling, which can be said to be the Aura of the thought. In short, feeling creates thoughts. So in deep meditation you are effortlessly fixed to a feeling which is the creator of thoughts. This is the expansion of our awareness or consciousness and not contraction of the same.

In our day to day thinking process, a thought, much like an Aura, has a feeling contained in and surrounding it, but this feeling is heavily limited, formed and constricted. In deep meditation, the feeling we experience is unbound, unobstructed and in its purest nature. In short, deep meditation reveals more clearly the feeling, rather than the logical thought.

When we think or concentrate on a thought, the very nature of concentration limits or make us unable of the feeling. Therefore it is necessary to move from concentration to meditation. In concentration we are unable to go beyond thoughts because of our hardened mental habits which keep us away from creativity, habits which keep our mind in a continuous rut. Thus meditation assists in developing the sensitivity of feeling awareness and this breaks the hardened habits of the past, on each and every level of our being. This increases our sensitivity relating to objects, thoughts etc. Hence meditation is being aware in the state of feeling, and one should not confuse this feeling with emotions. There is an important difference. Emotions are sharp energies that force us into physical or mental activity whereas feeling is awareness without any compulsion behind it.

In meditation, there are no thoughts; if there are thoughts or we are thinking then we are concentrating and not meditating. Although, meditation is a state of feeling, it is very difficult to sustain that state for a long time. This state can be maintained for a very short time, a few seconds. In the feeling-state of meditation, the meditator, the object of meditation and the process of meditation becomes one and therefore in meditation there is a definite feeling of bliss. Wisdom or knowledge is the strength of the mind. Once we are deep into meditation we must realize what is happening in consciousness and become aware of meaningfulness with that meditation. Because of the functioning of the super intelligence, the meditator feels and comes to know the indwelling meditator or the 'Self'. It is the enfoldment of understanding, dignity, maturity and compassion. When we arrive at this state, ignorance is transcended.

This state of pure feeling or non-thinking state of meditation is a very powerful state. It is not an unconscious, illogical or an abstract state, it is a living experience. The thoughts in concentration are gross while the feelings in meditation are subtle.

Beyond meditation exists the Super Subtlest State called the Samadhi.

Helpline to Practice Meditation

1) **Meditation Area:** A place should be set aside for the purpose of meditation. The room in which the place is set should not be stuffy and the furnishing should be as simple as possible, without cluttering. The room should not be totally dark but there should be medium light, enough to distinguish various objects in the room. The temperature of the room should be comfortable for us. Cold hands and feet are not conducive to meditation.
There should be peaceful vibrations in the room and we should have a feel-good factor when we enter the room.

2) **Silence:** Music should not be played during meditation, the noise level should be reduced and external attractions should be minimum.

3) **Incense:** A lightly scented sandalwood incense or flower fragrance may be used.

4) **Meditation mat:** A woolen blanket, a flannel cloth or a silk cloth should be sat upon. They are good conductors and do not allow the powerful cosmic vibrations you acquire during meditation to be grounded, or, earthing does not take place.

5) **Vibrations:** The practice of asanas and other exercises should not be done in the same place that we meditate, as the vibrations set up are often contradictory.

6) **Clothing:** The clothes should be loose and comfortable and should not be sticking to the body.

7) **Posture:** We may use any meditative posture for meditation in which we feel comfortable, taking care that the spine is erect, neck parallel to the floor and the body totally relaxed.

8) **Dietary habits:** Meditation should be practiced neither on a full stomach nor in a state of hunger. Leave a gap of 2 to 4 hours after a full meal before we begin meditation.

9) **Direction:** During the day we should meditate facing **east**, in the direction of the rising sun and in the evening after the sun sets, we should face **north** in the direction of the Polar star.

10) **Eye Position:** We should concentrate at the Ajna chakra or the 3rd eye i.e. eyes are closed and gently focused at the root of the nose in between the eyebrows. Do not stare but gently gaze. There should be no strain on your eyes.

11) **Best Time:** The best time for meditation is 4 a.m. to 6 a.m. early morning as it is said to be the Brahma Mahurat. At this time there are balanced energies and they are strongest. Second best time is after sun set 6 p.m. to 8 p.m. in the evening.

Apart from these two timings you can meditate at any time, for any time is a great time. **Meditate every day.** Make an effort to select a convenient time when we can consistently and regularly meditate. The habit of meditating each day regularly, at the same time, same place and in the same way is extremely valuable in establishing overall discipline and control of the Cosmic energy and thus our mind.

Guidelines for Meditation for Beginners

1) The feeling is a very important and prominent factor in meditation. Our 'object' of meditation should be such that it produces a pleasant feeling, a

feeling of unselfish love. Our feeling should be to give of ourselves of what we are and without thinking of what we will get in return or without any thought of rewards. We should strive for such a feeling in meditation.

2) A very important point is that, we should understand that it is the nature of the mind to wander, so in meditation the mind is bound to jump from one thought to another. Therefore we should not make the mistake of getting upset when the mind wanders because the mind energies are very much scattered when we get emotional. We should not be bothered if we have to bring the mind to the focus of the object of meditation any number of times. Gently focusing the mind without being disturbed will soon bring success in meditation. With a little practice and a little patience the mind will become focused on the object of meditation without deviation and will be well disciplined.

3) After we finish our meditation, sit quietly for some time and introspect the cause of interference which made the mind wander. This will help us to release and neutralize this energy of interference and prevent it from disturbing us in future. Secondly give more importance to the object of meditation; this will help us to overcome the interference.

4) Beginners should remember that it is the quality that matters and not the quantity. Beginners make the mistake of making the effort to sit for too long a period. It is always better to sit for a short time in a joyous, comfortable state than strain ourselves unnecessarily and try to meditate for an hour or so. Start the practice with 15 to 20 minutes and slowly increase the time of meditation. When the mind starts wandering, either bring it back gently to the object of meditation or understand now it is the time to stop meditation and practice it again later.

5) Practice meditation regularly and first form a habit. By regular practice at fixed time and place, our mind gets conditioned and accepts easily and remains silent or wandering becomes less. This makes meditation a joyous experience and it becomes automatic and effortless. Thus the mind remains pleasant and can focus on the object of meditation rather than on the process of meditation.

6) Some time it could happen that our mind is particularly disturbed or if we are physically sick, it is suggested that we maintain the practice of sitting in meditation at the fixed time and place. Though we may not be meditating yet we hold on to the habit and also understand that we are not breaking the regular pattern of daily meditation which will give us an inner satisfaction.

7) It is observed that beginners, after some time of practice, become impatient. We start expecting to get results or some experiences and when we fail to get them, we start wandering: 'Am I doing it right? Were my hands placed right and my body still?' etc.etc. so this shows that instead of focusing on the object of meditation we are focusing on the process. In the beginning stages of meditation, the enfoldment is not rapid. Meditate for the enjoyment and the feeling that meditation gives and not to accomplish anything. Do not expect the result so fast. Remember every action has got a reaction, someday we will definitely succeed.

8) First we must be patient and take our own time to understand and properly grasp each stage and the meaning of the technique of meditation, only then we can meditate with a proper attitude. When proper attitude is established then the spiritual progress is faster. Some may take months even to start the right way of meditation and some may advance faster; it all depends on our attitude and understanding.

9) It is very difficult to judge the true inner depth of our meditation, so it is useless to worry how much we have progressed. Without being disheartened we must continue the search within, for meditation is the search within the heart of a soul. It is easier to judge others than our own self so other people will find the natural change, the maturity in us long before we discover it ourselves. So we should be patient and regular in our practice and one day success will definitely be ours.

10) Meditation is a process of moving from the outer physical world of impermanence to the inner spiritual world, the search for reality, our inner 'Real Self'. So practice regularly and patiently and we will one day achieve great joy, peace and bliss.

Actual Practice of Meditation

1) Sit comfortably on the asana, spine erect, head straight and body completely relaxed and the eyes focused on the Ajna chakra or 3rd eye.

Start with Sahaja Pranayama

When we practice Pranayama before meditation it helps us to collect our spread-out attention and awareness and it brings to a focal point. Thus Pranayama helps us to concentrate during meditation. Secondly, before we start any auspicious work we always pray first to Lord Ganapati or Vinayaka who is the presiding deity of Pranayama and is therefore called Pranavaswaroopa.

Actual Practice of Sahaja Pranayama: Start with left nostril, inhale counting 3 – hold for 12 counts – exhale counting 6. Ratio is 1:4:2. Again inhale from the right nostril and hold counting 12, exhale counting 6. This is **one round. Six** such rounds makes **one cycle.**

Practice minimum 2 rounds and maximum as much as we are comfortable with, before meditation. We should increase the counts and rounds with practice.

Note: One may refer Chapter 5 Pranayama for more details.

2) **The second step is PRAYERS:**

Prayer is a direct, **one-to-one link with God**. It is our **own feelings expressed in words**. The prayer creates **a rapport** between us and God.

Baba says:

"There are two roads to fulfillment; prayer and meditation. Prayer makes you a supplicant at the feet of God; *dhyana* **(meditation) induces God to come down to you and inspires you raise yourselves to Him. It tends to make you come together, not place one in a lower level and the other on a higher."**

SSS Vol. V 'Lamps Lit from the Same Flame'

The easiest way to have a direct link with God is pray as soon as we get up in the morning, on the bed itself. Remember: Every **night we die and every morning we are born again.** So we should **thank Him for the day and request Him to function through you.**

Ex. **Morning Prayer:** "Oh! God I thank you for showing me this day. Be with me throughout the day.

1) Breathe through me, 2) think through me, 3) see through me,4) hear through me, 5) smell through me, 6) touch through me,7) speak through me,8) eat through me, 9) work through me,10) walk through me and 11) feel through me. Do all my activities in thoughts words and deeds through me. I pray to Thee for Thy Presence with me throughout the day."

After praying in the morning, please do not leave God at the altar and go and start the work. Take Him along with us in all that we do, say in the kitchen or in the office etc. Initially imagine that He is by our side all the time. Slowly we will start experiencing His presence. In this way we can have a very fast and direct link with God.

Meditation Prayer: Before meditation it is necessary to connect ourselves with Him i.e. our God or Guru because it is **impossible for us to achieve the goal of self-realization without Him.** So we can have our own prayer (speak to God). For ex.

"I pray to Thee Oh! Lord to guide me in all walks of life, especially on my spiritual path. Guide me from ignorance to knowledge, darkness to light, restlessness to restfulness, peace and bliss. Fill my heart with immense Love and devotion. Guide me till I merge in Thy Pure Consciousness forever and ever to be free from the cycle of birth and death forever and ever. Please be with me throughout, GUIDE ME and PROTECT ME, SHOWER THY GRACE and BLESSING UPON ME, Oh! Lord Sai".

So prayer puts us in direct link with God and when we **pray sincerely from the core of our Heart, God definitely responds.** Just as we pray before meditation we should say a prayer of **THANKSGIVING** after meditation.

THANKSGIVING PRAYER: "I thank you Oh! Lord for the guidance and pray to thee to BE with me through out."

Prayer is also **one of the ways of showing Love and Gratitude towards God or Guru for all that He has been doing for us.**

Night Prayer: Pray at night before going to bed and offer everything at His Lotus Feet.

"Oh! Lord, all the Karmas or actions that I have done throughout the day, in thoughts, words, and deeds, I surrender at Thy Lotus Feet. I am not bound by any of these Karmas as I am not the body, I am not the mind and I am not the intellect. I am Pure Consciousness. Swami Please be with me throughout the night."

So regularly pray:

1) **Morning Prayer as soon as we get up.**
2) **Before having our food or we eat anything, offer it to the Lord.**
3) **Before Meditation –After meditation.**
4) **Before we go to bed.**

3) The third step is SAVITRI PRANAYAMA

We i.e. our body, mind and soul is a miniature of the entire Creation. Whatever is there in the entire Universe is also present in our body. **Pinda or Microcosm is a part of Brahmand or Macrocosm.**

i.e. a drop of sea water has all the qualities of the sea.

As Brahmand or Macrocosm has different levels or states of consciousness similarly our Pinda or Microcosm too has the same levels of Consciousness.

The different levels of consciousness are in the 7 Chakras or energy centers (they are also known as the 7 worlds or Sapta Lokas) and are as follows:

Muladhara - Bhu, Swadhistan - Bhuvah, Manipur - Suvah, Anahat - Maha, Vishudha - Jana, Ajna - Tapa, Sahasrara - Satyam.

For deep concentration we have **to collect our consciousness / awareness** which is encaged and spread in our entire body and bring it to Ajna Chakra. As Consciousness is every where it requires a vehicle to be carried; so Pranava or Om is the vehicle. So we lift our consciousness from one conscious level to another with the help of Pranava or Om which is called the **SAVITRI MANTRA.**

Besides the Gayatri maha – mantra, Vedas have given another great mantra, **SAVITRI MANTRA** which is a magic formula to achieve highest state of consciousness in meditation.

PRACTICE: (This practice is repeated here for your convenience).

Take our awareness from feet to the 3rd Eye or Ajna chakra each time chant Om Bhu i.e. Start with chanting Om at the same time lifting up our awareness slowly and when it reaches the Ajna chakra chant Bhu. Repeat this 5 times. While carrying our awareness from the feet, take a pause at the Muladhar chakra for a second and then move ahead towards Ajna chakra. Continue the process as follows:

OM from feet to MULADHAR to AJNA- - - -Bhu - 5 times

OM from feet to SWADHISTAN - AJNA ————Bhuva - 5 times

OM from feet to MANIPUR - AJNA ————Suvah - 5 times

OM from feet to ANAHAT - AJNA ————Maha - 5 times

OM from feet to VISHUDHA - AJNA————Jana - 5 times

OM from feet to AJNA - AJNA ————Tapa - 5 times

OM from feet to AJNA - SAHASRATA Satyam – 5 times.

Note: The reader can also refer Savitri Pranayama in Chapter No. 5 – Pranayama.

4) The fourth step is SOHAM:

What is Soham?

Soham is our very breath, the life principle without which we cannot live. If we minutely observe, we will realize that when we inhale air, the sound created by our breath is 'SO' which means 'I' and when we exhale air, the sound created is 'HAM' which means 'HE'.

The breath is reminding us of our identity with the Supreme Soul. We breathe 21,600 times daily @ 15 Sohams or complete breaths per minute approx.

Soham should be done by **consciously** watching the incoming and outgoing breath and mentally associating ourselves with attributes of divinity, like peace, Love, purity, bliss etc. in meditation.

Swami says:

"Man breathes at the rate of 900 times per hour, 21,600 times per day i.e. 10800 times during day time. With every breath man is supposed to repeat 'SOHAM' ['I am He'], so the figure 216 and its half, 108 has a deep significance. It is also 9 times 12; 9 being the number indicative of BRAHMAN, since it is always nine, however many times you may multiply it (9x12=108, 1x9=9, 9x9=81, 8+1=9) and 12 is the number of SUNS; also the SUN moves through 12 points, each representing 1 month, just as 9 is the symbol of BRAHMAN, 8 is the number of MAYA"

SSS: Vol. IV: Page 228 (25 Nov.64)

Explaining the technique of advanced meditation on Soham, Bhagavan Baba says:

"With each breath, you are averring 'Soham', I am He. Not only you, every being avers it. It is a fact which you have ignored so long. Believe it now. When you watch your breath and meditate on that grand Truth, slowly the 'I' and the 'He' will merge and there will no more be two, for Soham will be transformed into Om. The Primal sound, Pranava which the Vedas proclaim as the symbol of the Nirakara Para Brahman. That Om is the swa-swaroopa, the Reality behind all this relative unreality"

Sai Baba and Moksha – By P.P.Arya, P. 38

Hence **SOHAM** is a very useful technique to help us to concentrate. Practice Soham for about 7 to 10 minutes or till our thoughts have reduced and then start with **Concentration.** Continue focusing at the Ajna Chakra on the image of our God or Guru or on any object of concentration which gives us contentment. Initially our mind may wander but with a little patience and practice it will start focusing. Continue the practice for 15 to 20 minutes to start with then increase the time. When we are through with our meditation say the **thanksgiving prayer** (mentioned above) take 2 long deep breaths and slowly open the eyes and come out of meditation.

Bhagwan Baba has given the following procedure of Dhyana:

"First when you sit for meditation, repeat a few shlokaas on the glory of God so that the agitated mind may be calmed. Then gradually, while doing Japa visualize the form which the name represents. When your mind wanders away from the form, lead it onto the name. Let it dwell on the sweetness of either the name or the form. Thus, the turbulent mind can be easily tamed." "The imaginary form you have visualized will gradually get transmuted into the Bhaava Chithra dear to the heart and fixed in the memory. As one progresses, it will become the Saakshaatkaara Chithra – vision of the actual form when the Lord assumes that form in order to fulfill your aspiration. This Saadhhana is called Japasahitha dhhyaana or meditation with recitation of the name. I advise you all to take it up for it is the best form of dhhyaana, especially for beginners."

"Within a few days, you will taste the joy of meditation. After about ten or fifteen minutes of this dhhyaana in the initial stages, and longer periods after some time, do manana or contemplation on the shaanthi and aanandha which you enjoyed during the dhyaana,"

A check list for easy reference:

1) Sahaja Pranayama
2) Prayers for guidance and protection, grace and blessings.
3) Savitri Pranayama or technique
4) Soham
5) Concentration and Meditation
6) Thanksgiving Prayer
7) Two deep breaths and coming out of meditation.

We have now studied in details all about meditation. When we practice meditation sincerely and regularly, it slowly culminates into a higher stage called Samadhi or equipoise. Let us discuss Samadhi in our next Chapter.

SAI RAM

'Samadhi'

"Samadhi is a state of equal-mindedness. It is the state in which the oneness of everything is experienced".

– Sri Satya Sai Baba

Chapter VIII
Samadhi or Equipoise

WHAT IS SAMADHI

The sincere and regular practice of meditation will slowly lead to the 8th stage of Sai Astang Yoga i.e. **SAMADHI**. 'Dhi' means Buddhi and sama means equal i.e. Samadhi means equal mindedness. At this stage, one's identity becomes both externally and internally immersed in meditation. The meditator, the act of meditation and the object meditated upon, all three shed their individual characteristics and merge with one single vision of the entire cosmos. **Samadhi means complete absorption in the self.** The person in this state is always in blissful awareness of the self. He experiences pleasure and pain, happiness and sorrow, with equanimity; in short we go beyond duality and experience oneness with the entire cosmos.

In the state of Samadhi we realizes that we are not the body, mind or the Ego sense which is transitory and impermanent but becomes aware of the truth and reality that 'I' is pure consciousness, a pure formless state. One understands that truth has no beginning and it has no end and that it has existed both inside and outside of one's self eternity. There is the realization that we are, we were and we shall always be the truth i.e. Pure Consciousness.

In Samadhi we experiences tranquility and calm passivity. In this state we are free of time and space element and hence free of karmas as karmas exist only in the realm of time and space. We are free from all cravings of things, and experiences peace and bliss at all times. Hence Samadhi is neither a state of physical unconsciousness nor a lethargic state of nonexistence, but a complete state of awareness or consciousness.

The bondage that is so much talked about is internal and not external. It is our very mind that binds us to the earth plane. So the mind should be freed, only then can we experience the real freedom.

Who is Seeking Freedom or Liberation?

The actual meaning of freeing the mind means giving up the doership or the false 'I' or Ego. Once we realize that we are not the body and mind then the question arises, Who am I? Who is doing all the actions? And we realizes that all our actions, physical as well as mental are but the conditioning of the mind of our past happenings. So actions just happen and if actions are just happening than who is this 'I'?

In actuality the 'I' or Ego does not exist and its 'existence' is merely a matter of divine will or divine hypnosis, and that our notion of free will is based on the programming in the body-mind organism- genes plus environmental conditioning- over which the ego or 'I' has had no control.

The Ego or I has to convince itself that every single action has been based on some prior happening, over which it has no control from his personal investigation into his personal experiences then **it is finally compelled to SURRENDER ITS SENSE OF PERSONAL DOERSHIP**, and no one is doer of any action, neither himself nor the 'other, that all that happens at any moment, through any body- mind organism is brought about by the **primal Energy functioning through each body-mind organism according to GOD'S WILL OR COSMIC LAW.**

Thus when the ego or the false 'I' surrenders its doership and accepts that everything happens as per God's will, only then one attains Freedom or Liberation.

In Samadhi, the perception is instantaneous. The ultimate experience is a matter of milli-seconds of time when there is oneness between the meditator, the object of meditation and the process of meditation, or rather it occurs when the mind becomes one with the object and one obtains direct experience of the divine illumination, which is indeed a precious gift from the Eternal Lord.

In this experience of Samadhi, the mind no longer remains as an internal thinking instrument but is completely merged or unified with the consciousness. As long as the state of Samadhi lasts we will have this heightened awareness and when the Samadhi ends, it remains in the memory track of our being, never to be lost or forgotten.

It is also said that Samadhi is the blending of individual Consciousness into the Pure Eternal Consciousness.

Types of Samadhi

There are different stages of Samadhi explained with various names such as Sa-Vitarka, Nir-Vitarka, Nir-vichar, Asmita etc. But broadly speaking there are **2 types of Samadhis; Savikalpa Samadhi and Nirvikalpa Samadhi.**

1) **SAVIKALPA SAMADHI**

    Complete absorption of the mind in the Divine, like the river merging in the ocean. According to my God and Guru Bhagwan Sri Satya Sai Baba, Savikalpa Samadhi is a state where the aspirant retains his individual identity while experiencing the Divine. In this Samadhi there is Duality or Dhwaitha Bhava.

2) **NIRVIKALPA SAMADHI**

    Complete absorption of the mind in the Divine, including his individual identity. In this Samadhi one loses the individual identity completely. There is no duality and one experiences complete oneness with the Divine.

When a person attains the Samadhi state there is a great change in his character and behavior. Samadhi bestows **Sama-buddhi** that is complete equanimity in one's life. The person becomes more introverted, speaks less is contented and free of all cravings, free of all tensions and worries, is always in the present, and always functions from the divine or conscious level.

REVISION OF THE 5 GROSS STATES

1) *1ˢᵗ State: Jagrutha Avastha or the Wakful State:*

   As we are experiencing earth life, we have become aware that we exist. We become aware of the mind- body instrument which makes us aware that we exist. The struggle we face within this existence makes us understand what life is all about and that we are alive. With this self awareness we start our inward path towards consciousness.

2) *2ⁿᵈ State: Pratyahara or Sense Withdrawal:*

   In the second state, we move inwards to the mental realm, freeing ourselves of the gross material world. In this state, there is sense-withdrawal, which is initially a very slow process but later we begin to have control over our internal and external life.

3) *3ʳᵈ State: Dharana or Concentration:*

   In the third state, we try to eliminate all our other mental patterns and focus our attention of the one mental object of concentration. We hold on to this object of concentration with effort and in the process transcend the mental realm without transcending the object of concentration. This is the third step towards self realization or liberation.

4) *4ᵗʰ State: Dhyana or Meditation:*

   In this state we hold on to the object of concentration with less effort and slowly we hold it effortlessly. The process of meditation has started. As we progress in meditation the object of meditation starts dissolving into our consciousness and our consciousness into the object. Hence meditation happens when the meditator, meditation and the process of meditation become one.

5) *5ᵗʰ State: Samadhi:*

   This is a state of heighten meditation. In Sanskrit this state is called Vritti-Nirodha. Vritti means mind-activity and nirodha means stopping or holding. This is the state when the last final object in our mind is dropped and now the mind is in its pure unformed state. Individual consciousness has now become Universal consciousness. This is a supra conscious state.

In this state the self beholds the self which is the truth of reality principle. This state in Sanskrit is called as 'Aham-brahmasmi' which means I am the Brahman. It is at this point Samadhi is attained.

Supreme happiness, free from pleasure, pain or misery is experienced. **Samadhi is the climax of Dhyana.**

SAI RAM

'Surrender'

"If you have firm faith in God and surrender to His Will,
He will not fail you.

The Bliss that can be derived from this surrender to God cannot
be got through any other means".

– Sri Satya Sai Baba

The Conclusion

The journey on the pathway to self-realization attains fulfillment only when we sincerely, regularly and strictly follow all the eight steps of Sai Asthang Yoga and we ultimately reach our destination.

In our day-to-day life we should practice steps one to six, that is Yama, Niyama, Asanas, Pranayama, Pratyahar and Dharana. When practicing Dharana or concentration we glide into meditation which ultimately culminates into Samadhi.

Yama: The Shad Ripus; Kama, Krodha, Lobha, Moha, Madh and Matshar are to be strictly avoided. When we practice ceiling on desires, the shad ripus are automatically controlled. The Niyama: Sathya, Dharma, Shanti, Prema and Ahimsa are to be firmly observed. When Yama and Niyama become part of our life there comes a definite change in our thought patterns, which naturally brings a positive change in our attitude. This has a tremendous effect on our physical and mental health.

Next comes the practice of Asanas. When practiced regularly, they make the body supple and healthy; this prepares the body for further deeper practices on the path of Sai Ashtang Yoga. The body becomes fit for sitting for many hours in concentration and meditation.

The practice of Pranayama is of utmost important as it helps to control the life-force or Prana. The regular practice of Pranayama not only keeps us physically healthy by keeping us free of major diseases, but also keeps us full of energy or Prana, and steadies our mind, which is very important in the practice of both Pratyahar, or sense control and Dharana, or concentration.

Our monkey mind, which is very difficult to control, becomes submissive with the practice of Pranayama, and is more easily controlled. This helps to steady the mind for concentration.

When the above four outer steps of Yama, Niyama, Asana and Pranayam are sincerely and regularly followed, then the next four inner or subtler steps of Pratyahar, Dharana, Dhyana and Samadhi become easy to follow.

It is difficult to concentrate when the mind is distracted. As concentration is not a mental condition but a function of the mind, we should consciously make effort to focus our mind and concentrate. Just thinking becomes a distraction to learning. So a distracted mind cannot learn to concentrate and without concentration we can never free our mind. Hence with the above-mentioned practices of Pranayama and Pratyahar we can free the mind from distraction.

Our mind is ruled by the trigunas of Sattva or equanimity, Rajas or hyper activity and Tamas or dullness or lethargy. To attain spiritual insight, our mind should be ruled by Sattva or equanimity. In this state of Sattva, the mind unfolds, and is serene, collected and wise. Through deep concentration, this state of sattva can be attained.

In the Chapter, 'Dharana' or concentration; various techniques were mentioned, especially the visualization technique, the 'Who am I' and the Tratak, all of which which are very useful and accelerate the process of concentration.

The practice of Dharana or concentration, helps us to remove the physical and mental imbalances of our modern day lifestyle. This effort is reciprocal, for as we learn to concentrate and gain success in Yoga, our life will become more balanced and meaningful. When concentration is practiced sincerely and regularly it evolves into meditation. Meditation happens when our mind is trained to focus, and is able to sustain this focus of attention through concentration (Dharana) unbounded by time and space.

We must always remember the three fundamental basic requirements for an aspirant or disciple to reach the goal of self realization. They are:

1) **Immense love for God**
2) **Purity of mind**
3) **Attitude of complete self surrender.**

With these three powerful tools, one is very much inspired to sit for the practice of meditation, which is most required, especially in the initial stages.

Continuous repetition of the Lord's name (Japa) along with the practice of Yama and Niyama will bring purity of mind, and the mind and intelligence will be cleansed and tamed to concentrate (Dharana) and thus be prepared for Meditation.

Meditation cannot be taught, it just happens when we tread the inward path through Dharana or concentration and focus and sustain one-pointed attention on the image of our God or Guru along with Japa. When we are able to focus with one-pointed attention, then the mind is said to be contemplating. As the mind contemplates, it slowly glides into meditation. In meditation there is no effort involved, it is an effortless, deep quietude of the mind.

The entire process of concentration, contemplation and meditation seem like separate movements but they occur or happen simultaneously when we sit for the practice of concentration.

When we thus meditate effortlessly, the calmness and quietude is the link between meditation and Samadhi. Samadhi is a heightened state, where thought is transcended and we ascend towards spiritual consciousness.

Samadhi is the highest state where we lose body consciousness, completely transcend the thought or mind or the ego sense and become aware of the truth and reality of the 'I', where there is only the feeling of existence or pure awareness or pure consciousness: a pure formless state. There is a realization that we always existed without beginning or end, in eternity, as Truth, as pure Consciousness.

To put this feeling in beautiful words 'It is as if God carries us in His arms like a small innocent carefree baby, through eternity. In fact, there is no duality at all. 'God' and 'us' are not separate, but two moving as one in eternity'. Such a state is difficult to express in words. It can only be experienced.

My best wishes to all readers and spiritual seekers. May this book 'Sai Ashtang Yoga' be an inspiring and guiding force to you all. May you attain ultimate peace and bliss. May Sai bless you all.

SAI RAM

References

- Anonymous, **Bases of Sadhana**. Compiled from Divine Discourses of Bhagawan Sri Sathya Sai Baba.

- Anonymous, (July, 2002). **Towards Human Excellence, Book 2, The Five Human Values**. Sri Sathya Sai EHV Trust, Institute of Sathya Sai Education, Mumbai.

- Anonymous, (June 2008). **Education in Human Values, A Coursebook for Training of Master Trainers**. Lt. Col.G.C.Khosla on behalf of Sri Sathya Sai International Centre for Human Values, **Delhi**.

- Anonymous, (July 2006). **Towards Human Excellence, Book 9, Inspiring Stories**. Institute of Sathya Sai Education, Mumbai,

- Bhagawan Sri Sathya Sai Baba, (January 1999). **Dhyana Vahini**. Sri Sathya Sai Books & Publication Trust, Prashanti Nilayam, India.

- B.N. Narasimha Murthy, (2006). **Helpline on the Sathya Sai Path** (compiled by Dr. Kaushik Narayan). Sri Sathya Sai Publication Society, Kerala.

- Goswami Kriyananda, (March 1976). **The Spiritual Science of Kriya Yoga**, Temple of Kriya Yoga, Chicago, U.S.A.

- Paramhansa Nityananda, (December 2005). **Beyond Life and Death**. Nityananda Vedic Science University Press, Nityananda Vedic Science University, U.S.A.

- Swami Atmatattwananda Saraswati, **Steps to Raja Yoga**. Satyam Prakashan, Satya Darshan Ashram, Rishikesh, India.

- Swami Sathyanand Saraswati, (1993). **Asana Pranayama Mudra Bandha**. Sri G.K. Kejriwal, Hon. Secretary, Bihar School of Yoga, Ganga Darshan, Munger, Bihar, India

About the Author

Dr. Kavita Bhatt has graduated in Psychology; she is a Naturopath and has completed M.D. in Alternative Medicines.

She has completed many Healing courses. She is a Reiki Grand Master, Advanced Pranic Healer, Astrologer, Gemologist, Palmist, Face Reader, Aura Reading and Past Life Regression. She has also practiced Crystal Therapy, Pendulum Therapy, Pyramid Therapy etc.

She is an author of 5 books with her Guru's guidance. The names of the books are:

1) 'Sai Ashtang Yoga'
2) 'My Sai and I'
3) 'The Sea of Sai Consciousness'
4) 'Sai –The Source of all Energies Baba - The Ultimate Consciousness'
5) 'The Soul's spiritual Journey from Reflection to Reality'
6) 'The teachings of Sanatan Dharma'- From teachings of Vasistha Yoga to teaching of Sri Sathya Sai Baba – Sanatan Dharma continues ….. will soon be released.

At present she is holding Meditation Camps, Pranayam Camps, Giving Presentations, Talks and Study Circles at various places in Mumbai and also in various other states of India.

At present she is treating patients as Free Service, following the Divine guidance of her Guru Sri Sathya Sai Baba. She does counseling and treats patients with flower remedies, treating the mind which helps in healing the body.

SAI RAM